# Diagnosis and Management of Rhinitis

First Edition

## *William Wagner, MD*
Head, Section of Allergy and Immunology,
Department of Pulmonary and
Critical Care Medicine,
Clevelend Clinic Foundation,
Cleveland, Ohio

## *Mani S. Kavuru, MD*
Director, Pulmonary Function Laboratory,
Department of Pulmonary
and Critical Care Medicine,
Cleveland Clinic Foundation,
Cleveland, Ohio

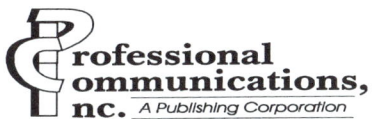

**Copyright 1996**
William Wagner, MD
and Mani S. Kavuru, MD
Cleveland, Ohio

*Published by:*
**Professional Communications, Inc.**

All rights reserved. No part of this publication may be reproduced or transmitted in any form or by any means, electronic or mechanical, including photocopy, recording or any other information storage and retrieval system, without the prior agreement and written permission of the publisher. Requests for permission or further information should be addressed to Professional Communications, Inc.; P.O. Box 10; Caddo, OK 74729-0010; or faxed to 405/367-9989.

*For orders only, please call:*
**1-800-337-9838**

ISBN: 1-884735-02-9

Library of Congress Card Number: 96-067858

Printed in the United States of America

This text is printed on recycled paper.

# **DEDICATION**

To Jeanne, Brett, and Amanda

—**WW**

To Mom, Dad, and Joan

—**MSK**

# ACKNOWLEDGEMENTS

The authors wish to thank Rita Oppedisano and Patty Balas for preparation of the manuscript.

# TABBED TABLE OF CONTENTS

| | | |
|---|---|---|
| **Part 1**<br>*General Information* | Introduction | 1 |
| | Definition, Classification and Epidemiology | 2 |
| | Pathogenesis | 3 |
| **Part 2**<br>*Diagnosis of Rhinitis* | Diagnosis: History, Examination and Skin Testing | 4 |
| **Part 3**<br>*Therapy for Rhinitis* | Nonpharmacological Therapy | 5 |
| | Pharmacological Therapy | 6 |
| | Immunotherapy | 7 |
| **Part 4**<br>*References* | References | 8 |

# TABLES

| | | |
|---|---|---|
| Table 2.1 | Chronic Rhinitis Syndromes | 14 |
| Table 3.1 | Common Environmental Allergens by Season in the Northern United States. | 20 |
| Table 4.1 | Differential Diagnosis of Rhinitis | 30 |
| Table 5.1 | House-dust Mite Control Measures | 56 |
| Table 6.1 | Currently Available Pharmacologic Agents for Treatment of Rhinitis | 58 |
| Table 6.2 | Relative Efficacy of Drugs in Treatment of Rhinitis | 59 |
| Table 6.3 | Available $H_1$-Antihistamines | 60 |
| Table 6.4 | Decongestants | 66 |
| Table 6.5 | Steroid Nasal Inhalers | 70 |
| Table 6.6 | Relative Topical Vasoconstrictor Potency | 71 |
| Table 6.7 | Miscellaneous Agents for Rhinitis | 72 |
| Table 6.8 | Ocular Agents | 75 |
| Table 6.9 | Risk to Fetus of Allergy and Asthma Medications During Pregnancy | 76 |
| Table 6.10 | Risk of Allergy and Asthma Medications in First Trimester of Pregnancy | 77 |

# FIGURES

| | | |
|---|---|---|
| Figure 3.1 | Schematic of Nasal Mucosa: Immunologic Mechanisms Involved in Allergic Disease | 22 |
| Figure 3.2 | Summary of Proposed Mechanisms for Inflammation in Allergic Rhinitis | 23 |
| Color Plate 4.1 | Endoscopic View of a Nasal Polyp | 33 |

| | | |
|---|---|---|
| Color Plate 4.2 | Endoscopic View of Acute Purulent Sinusitis | 34 |
| Figure 4.1 | Overlap in Serum IgE Levels in Allergic Disease | 36 |
| Figure 4.2 | Normal Ostiomeatal Complex (Coronal View) | 38 |
| Figure 4.3 | Ostiomeatal Complex Obstruction and Secondary Sinusitis (Coronal View) | 39 |
| Figure 4.4 | Endoscopic View of Right Uncinate Process | 42 |
| Figure 4.5 | Simple CT of Normal Sinuses (Axial Views) | 43 |
| Figure 4.6 | Simple CT of Sinuses (Deviated Septum, No Sinusitis [Coronal View]) | 44 |
| Figure 4.7 | Simple CT of Sinuses Showing Extensive Bilateral Sinusitis (Axial View) | 45 |
| Figure 4.8 | Simple CT Demonstrates That the Left Maxillary Sinus Is Smaller, Without Sinusitis (Axial View) | 46 |
| Figure 4.9 | Plain X-ray Falsely Showing Opacification of Left Maxillary Sinus | 47 |
| Figure 4.10 | Simple CT Demonstrates a Large Left Maxillary Polyp Without Evidence of Sinusitis (Axial Views) | 48 |
| Figure 4.11 | Plain X-ray Showing Left Maxillary Opacification | 49 |
| Figure 4.12 | Plain X-ray Showing Air Fluid Level in the Left Maxillary Sinus | 50 |
| Figure 4.13 | Simple CT Demonstrates a Large Bony Spur of the Septum (Axial Views) | 51 |
| Figure 4.14 | Coronal CT Shows a Large Neuroblastoma Encroaching Into the Septum (Coronal View) | 52 |

# PART I

## GENERAL INFORMATION

# 1 Introduction

During the past decade, much has been learned about the inflammatory events of rhinitis. A diagnosis of rhinitis is based on history and physical findings correlated with allergy skin testing or *in vitro* testing. A detailed environmental history to identify the presence of external triggers is essential for both diagnosis and subsequent therapy. The goals of therapy for chronic rhinitis include:
- Restoration of nasal patency
- Control of nasal secretions
- Treatment of complications related to obstruction
- Prevention of recurrent symptoms

This text will review the pathogenesis, classification, differential diagnosis, clinical evaluation and overall management of rhinitis. Emphasis will be placed on recent developments, including pharmacologic advances.

# 2 Definition, Classification and Epidemiology

The common viral cold is probably the most common form of acute rhinitis. In addition to nasal symptoms, viral rhinitis has additional symptoms such as myalgia or sore throat and follows a predictable course of resolution within 10 days to 2 weeks. The patient with a "summer cold" lasting a full month is likely to have allergic rhinitis. Allergic rhinitis may also occur in an acute form, such as on direct contact with a cat or during the peak of an offending pollen season.

Most patients with allergic rhinitis have multiple inhalant sensitivities. The patient with pure ragweed allergic rhinitis is the exception rather than the rule. Allergic rhinitis is associated with allergen specific IgE and eosinophils in the nasal mucosa. Allergic rhinitis is by far the most common form of chronic rhinitis, occurring in perhaps 20 million people in the United States (7% to 10% of the population) and accounting for 3% of all office visits to physicians. A number of distinct disorders comprise the chronic rhinitis syndrome. The distinguishing features of these disorders are summarized in Table 2.1.

Anatomic contribution to chronic nasal congestion must be considered in all forms of chronic rhinitis. Nasal septal deformity may be congenital or acquired. The middle turbinates may be wider than normal due to the congenital presence of an air cell in the turbinate (concha bullosa). Nasal polyps are formed, but usually not until adult years (except in cystic fibrosis).

## TABLE 2.1 — CHRONIC RHINITIS SYNDROMES

| Symptom | Allergic Rhinitis | Vasomotor Instability | NARES* | Rhinitis Medicamentosa | Structural Rhinitis | Neutrophilic Rhinosinusitis | Polyps |
|---|---|---|---|---|---|---|---|
| Cause or mechanisms | Allergens hyperreactivity | Vascular | Unknown | Medication abnormalities | Septal | Infection | Inflammation |
| Sneezing and pruritus | +++ | – | ++++ | – | – | – | – |
| Rhinorrhea | +++ | ± | ++++ | – | – | Purulent | + |
| Congestion | ++ | ++++ | ± | +++ | +++ | ++ | ++++ |
| Postnasal drainage | + | ++++ | ± | – | – | +++ | ++ |
| Seasonal variation | Seasonal or perennial | Perennial | Perennial | Perennial | Perennial | Perennial | Perennial |
| Eosinophils in nasal secretion | + | – | + | – | – | – | + |
| Skin test results | Positive | Negative | Negative | Negative | Negative | Negative | Negative |

| Total IgE | Increased | Normal | Normal | Normal | Normal | Normal | Normal |
|---|---|---|---|---|---|---|---|
| Age at onset | Childhood | Adults | All ages | Adults | All ages | All ages | Adults |
| Associated factors | Family history, pale mucosa | Pregnancy, thyroid disorder | Pale mucosa | Use of topical decongestants, antihypertensives | Unilateral with obstruction; history of nasal trauma | Associated upper respiratory infection | Aspirin sensitivity |
| Treatment | Topical steroids, environmental control, immunotherapy | Decongestant, nasal saline, exercise | Topical steroids | Stop medication | Surgery | Antibiotics | Topical steroids, surgery |

* NARES = nonallergic rhinitis with eosinophilia syndrome

++++ = marked  ++ = mild  ± = questionable
+++ = moderate  + = slight  – = absent

Modified from: Slavin RG. Clinical disorders of the nose and their relationship to allergy. *Ann Allergy*. 1982;49:123.

Adenoid hypertrophy may obstruct the nasal passages of children and adolescents.

Some patients have hyperreactive noses responding with nasal congestion without allergic sensitization to nonspecific stimuli such as:
- Smoke
- Air pollution
- Odors

The term *vasomotor rhinitis* is used for this condition. These patients lack the itchy, watery eyes usually found along with an itchy, watery nose in allergic rhinitis/conjunctivitis. In fact, the absence of conjunctivitis casts doubt on a diagnosis of allergic rhinitis.

There is a condition known as *nonallergic rhinitis with eosinophilia syndrome* (NARES). In this condition, eosinophils are found in nasal secretions as in allergic rhinitis, but the patient does not have allergies. The same observation is frequently made in asthma; there may be abundant eosinophils in the bronchial secretions even though the patient does not have allergies.

Physicians must be aware that patients may affect their nasal condition for the worse by chronic use of decongestant sprays. An intermittent rhinitis may become a constant rhinitis (rhinitis medicamentosa) due to the rebound swelling between frequent doses of decongestant sprays. Severe nasal congestion may be associated with pregnancy. Birth control pills (pseudo pregnancy) occasionally cause nasal congestion. Hypothyroid patients may also experience nasal congestion.

The term *gustatory rhinitis* refers to rhinorrhea occurring during and after meals, usually seen in patients over age 60. Patients may suspect food allergy; but in these patients, food skin tests are negative and there is no preceding history of allergic rhinitis. The disorder seems to be due to nasal serous gland secretion at a time when there should be gastrointestinal gland secretion.

Disorders involving the nasal passages or the sinus cavities frequently accompany the symptoms of asthma. There is a substantial overlap between patients with asthma, rhinitis and nasal polyposis. Up to 50% to 80% of patients with asthma have rhinitis symptoms, whereas 10% to 15% of patients with perennial rhinitis have asthmatic symptoms. Methacholine responsiveness in the asthmatic range is seen in a significant number of patients with no overt history of asthma.

A study of 5,000 patients with asthma and/or allergic rhinitis reflects that 17% of asthmatics have nasal polyps, whereas 70% of patients with nasal polyps have asthma. Nasal polyps associated with rhinitis and asthma are seen primarily in patients who are over age 40. Asthmatic aspirin sensitivity is seen in over 30% of asthmatic patients with nasal polyps. Although aspirin sensitivity is not mediated by immunoglobulin E (IgE), aspirin may trigger severe asthma. Nasal polyps are at least twice as prevalent in rhinitis and asthma patients who have negative skin tests as those with positive skin tests. This suggests that nasal polyps are probably a manifestation, not of allergy, but of the underlying eosinophilic hypertrophic sinusitis that accompanies severe asthma and rhinitis. The only medications capable of shrinking polyps are topical and systemic corticosteroids. There appear to be a high incidence of radiographic sinus abnormalities in patients with asthma, perhaps over 50%.

# 3 Pathogenesis

The essential components of allergic reactions include:
- Allergens
- Immunoglobulin E (IgE) antibodies
- Mast cells
- Eosinophils

In allergic rhinitis, a complex inflammatory cascade results in the following pathophysiological hallmarks in the nasal mucosa and submucosa:
- Vasodilatation and edema formation
- Engorgement of mucous glands and goblet cells
- Infiltration of the submucosa and mucosa with eosinophils

This process results when inhaled allergens penetrate the nasal mucosal barrier (see Table 3.1 for a list of environmental allergens). Figure 3.1 is a schematic of the nasal mucosa. The antigen is processed by an antigen-presenting cell such as a macrophage, with subsequent activation of helper lymphocytes (probably $T_{H2}$ cells). Antigen specific IgE antibody is formed by plasma cells, which evolve from B-lymphocytes.

Figure 3.2 depicts a summary of proposed mechanisms for inflammation in allergic rhinitis. The isotype switch from B-lymphocyte production of immunoglobulin M (IgM) to production of IgE is promoted by interleukin 4 (IL-4), a $T_{H2}$ interleukin cytokine. Interleukin 5 (IL-5), another $T_{H2}$ cytokine, stimulates eosinophil production. Interleukins 3, 4 and 10 stimulate growth of mast cells. Thus the antibodies and cells needed for the allergic response are promoted by the

### TABLE 3.1 — COMMON ENVIRONMENTAL ALLERGENS BY SEASON IN THE NORTHERN UNITED STATES

| Season | Allergen |
| --- | --- |
| Early spring (February-May) | Tree pollens (elm, oak, hickory, maple) |
| Late spring (May-June) | Grasses (rye varieties) |
| Summer (July-August) | Ground or outdoor molds (*Alternaria, Fusarium, Cladosporium*) |
| Fall (mid-August–October) | Ragweed (plus cocklebur, lambs' quarter, pigweed, plantain) |
| Winter (November-February) and all year | Dust mites, animal emanations, cockroaches, molds (*Aspergillus, Alternaria, Penicillium*) |

Reproduced with permission from: Kaliner M, Lemanske R. Rhinitis and asthma. *JAMA*. 1992;268(20):2808.

cytokines of the $T_{H2}$ lymphocytes. Specific IgE binds to high-affinity receptors on the mast cell surface.

Bridging of two mast cell bound IgE molecules by allergen initiates mast cell degranulation with subsequent secretion of a variety of chemical mediators. Mediators released immediately are the preformed ones. These include:
- Histamine
- Eosinophil chemotactic factor
- Tryptase
- Chymase

Newly generated mediators are released within minutes of stimulation of the mast cells. These include:
- Products of metabolism of arachidonic acid

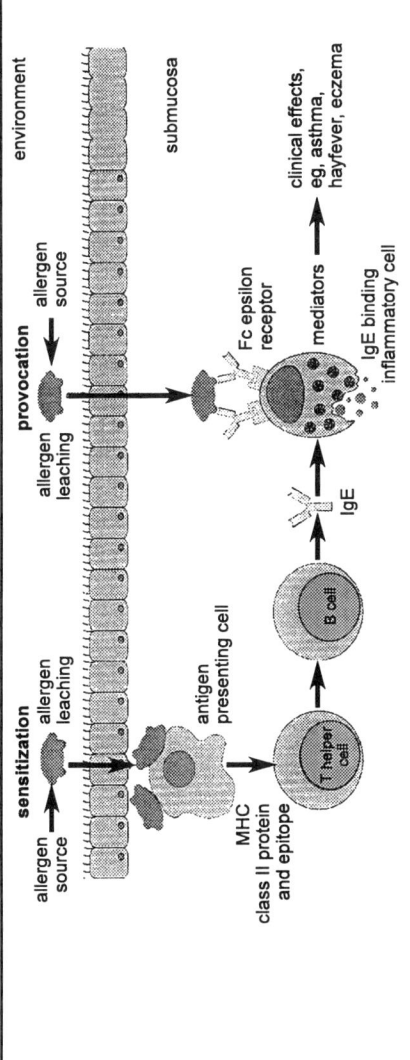

**FIGURE 3.1 — SCHEMATIC OF NASAL MUCOSA: IMMUNOLOGIC MECHANISMS INVOLVED IN ALLERGIC DISEASE**

Reproduced from: Holgate ST, Church MK. *Allergy*. London: Mosby; 1993:11.9.

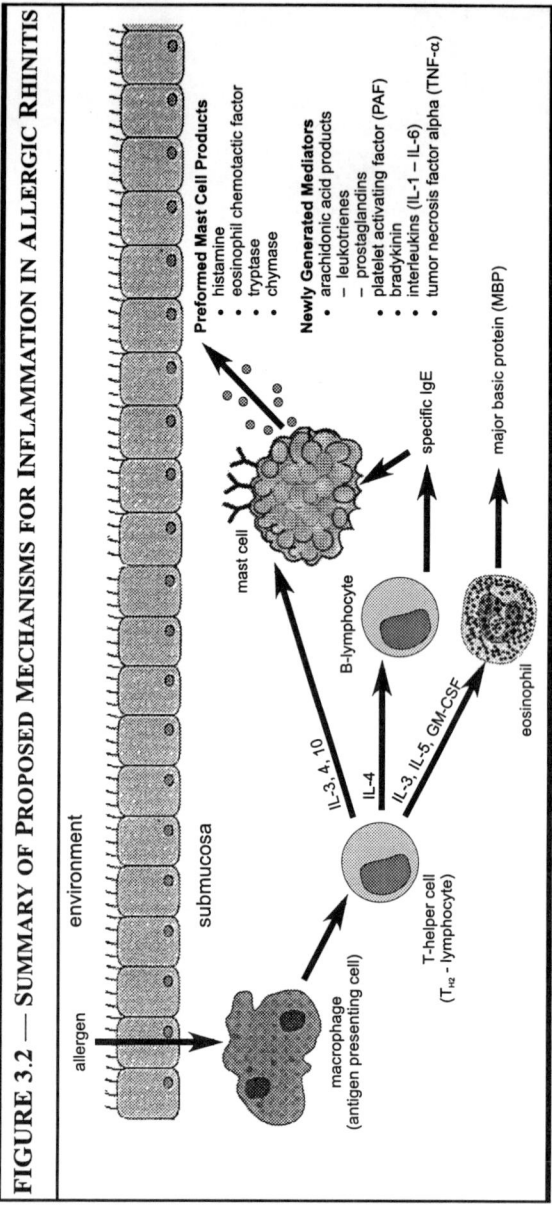

- Lipoxygenase — leukotrienes
- Cyclooxygenase — prostaglandins
• Platelet activating factor (PAF)
• Bradykinin
• Interleukins (IL-1 – IL-6)
• Tumor necrosis factor alpha (TNF-α)

Nasal itching is triggered by histamine and prostaglandins. Sneezing and rhinorrhea are triggered by histamine and leukotrienes. Nasal congestion is caused by histamine, kinins, leukotrienes and tumor necrosis factor alpha. The role of antihistamines and topical corticosteroids which inhibit the production of prostaglandins and leukotrienes in the symptomatic treatment of allergic rhinitis is well justified; but many mediators are involved, and the future may call for more antimediator therapies. Part of the appeal of immunotherapy is that the allergic response to environmental allergens is blunted and the release of mediators after allergen exposure is reduced.

The autonomic nervous system also makes a significant contribution to the pathogenesis of rhinitis. Nasal patency is greatly influenced by the sympathetic control of vascular tone. Rhinorrhea is under parasympathetic control. The peptide neurotransmitter (substance P) released from neurons may cause mast cell degranulation as well as directly affecting rhinorrhea and nasal congestion.

Many atopic individuals have biphasic responses to allergen challenge. The immediate response symptoms (such as itching, sneezing, rhinorrhea) and mediator levels return to baseline within 1 hour of allergen challenge. Without additional exposure to allergen, a patient with a late-phase response experiences a return of symptoms and a second rise in mediators at 3 to 11 hours after allergen challenge. Nasal congestion is the main symptom during the late-phase reaction. Pruritus is not prominent. Eosinophils characterize the mucosal infiltrate of the immediate allergic reaction. During the late phase, the eosinophils are joined by neutrophils and mononuclear cells. Corticosteroids, cromolyn sodium and immunotherapy reduce the severity of the late-phase reaction.

# PART 2

## Diagnosis of Rhinitis

# 4 Diagnosis: History, Examination and Skin Testing

The diagnosis of rhinitis is based on:
- History
- Physical examination
- Laboratory and skin testing

Allergic rhinitis and conjunctivitis usually develop in childhood or early adult years. Symptoms occasionally occur in response to ingested or injected allergens, but the vast majority of symptoms are in response to airborne allergens.

## History

Typical symptoms include:
- Sneezing
- Nasal pruritus
- Rhinorrhea with associated post-nasal drip
- Nasal congestion
- Itching and watering of the eyes
- Itching of the pharynx

Severe symptoms at peak seasons may interfere with sleep and cause fatigue. Loss of appetite may occur secondary to loss of the sense of smell. Headache is usually not a primary allergic symptom. Pain is usually not a primary allergic symptom. Recurrent chronic headache in the absence of sinusitis probably represents a second diagnosis, such as tension or vascular headache. The patient with allergic rhinitis may have a history of childhood eczema in the atopic dermatitis pattern of antecubital and popliteal distribution. First degree relatives often also have allergic rhinitis or asthma. A child who has a parent with allergic rhinitis has a 30% chance of having allergic rhinitis also. If both parents are affected, the chance of the child being atopic is in the range of 60%.

Consistent flare of symptoms around animals strongly suggests an allergic cause and is helpful in the diagnosis. The non-pet owner who is allergic to animal dander develops respiratory symptoms within minutes of contact with the animal or entering the house where the pet lives. The allergic patient may even react to the animal dander on the clothes of pet owners away from their homes. Prolonged daily exposure and persistence of animal allergens on the clothes prevent allergic pet owners from having abrupt changes in their symptoms when they enter or depart from their homes.

Interpretation of the significance of seasonal variation in symptoms is complex. Pollen seasons vary according to geographic location (see Table 3.1). In the Northeast and Midwest, tree pollen season begins in March and extends into June. Different trees pollinate in sequence, but many overlap. Willow and cottonwood release pollen in early spring; then maple peaks by mid-April, followed by birch in early May and oak in late May. In the Midwest, grass pollen reaches higher concentrations than in the Northeast and causes a significant allergic problem in June and July. Ragweed is the dominate pollen from mid-August to late September. In the Southeast, tree pollen emerges as early as mid-January. In the South, the northern grasses (timothy, blue grass, orchard grass, rye grass, and red top) are joined by the Bermuda grass; its antigens are not cross reactive with the northern grasses. In southern Florida, grass may pollinate year round. In the South Central region of the US, pecan joins the pollinating trees. On the West coast, olive is an important pollinating tree. Much of the West coast is free of ragweed.

The role of molds in allergic disease is not well understood. Mold spore counts may exceed pollen counts. Mold spores are in the air to some extent anytime the ground is not covered by snow. *Alternaria* and *Cladosporium* are among the most common outdoor mold spores found in the air. Mold spores may contribute to allergic rhinitis in the warm months of the year. A few patients will present with a consistent summer pattern of symptoms, yet have negative pollen and mold skin tests. Air temperature, humidity and air pollution may also contribute to a seasonal pattern of symptoms.

Perennial allergic rhinitis is more dependent on skin testing to establish the diagnosis. Symptoms fluctuate in severity, but recur throughout the year. Except in the deep South, pollen will disappear from the air for at least a month or two in the winter. However, indoor allergens are present year round. House-dust mites and animal danders are the most important of the indoor allergens currently known. Some patients with mite sensitivity may notice a flare of symptoms when dusting or using a vacuum cleaner.

Allergic rhinitis usually presents for the first time in a young person. Over 70% of patients with allergic rhinitis develop symptoms before age 30. Clinical allergic rhinitis usually subsides by the age of 50. Nasal symptoms developing for the first time after the age of 50 rarely have an allergic basis. Nasal polyps are a common cause of new, persistent nasal congestion in a middle-aged adult. A detailed environmental history to elicit the presence of external triggers is helpful for both diagnosis and subsequent avoidance therapy.

The differential diagnosis of rhinitis is shown in Table 4.1.

### TABLE 4.1—DIFFERENTIAL DIAGNOSIS OF RHINITIS

- Allergic
  - Seasonal (hay fever, rose fever)
  - Perennial
- Vasomotor
  - Perennial nonallergic
- Nonallergic rhinitis with eosinophils (NARES)
- Infectious
- Secondary rhinitis
  - Rhinitis medicamentosa
  - Pregnancy
  - Ciliary dyskinesia
  - Other local diseases
    - Polyps
    - Septal deviation
    - Tumor
    - Wegener granulomatosis
    - Foreign body

Modified from: Kaliner M, Lemenske R. Rhinitis and asthma. *JAMA*. 1992;268(20):2811.

## Physical Examination

It is important to realize that the allergic status of an individual is determined by the allergy history and allergy skin testing, not by examination of the nose. The physical examination of the nose detects the presence of anatomic factors, such as septal deviation or nasal polyps. The nasal speculum permits examination of the anterior nasal passages. In patients with chronic nasal obstruction, this view may be limited to little more than the nasal vestibule. Anterior nasal polyps may be visible using a nasal speculum.

Rhinoscopy using flexible or rigid endoscopes permits thorough examination of the nasal passages. This is particularly important in patients with the complication of chronic sinusitis. A rough idea of nasal patency may be obtained by asking the patient to inhale through the nose while gently occluding one nasal passage with pressure on the alar cartilage. If nasal obstruction on one or both sides is constant, an anatomic basis must be sought. Rhinoscopy provides the best means of physical diagnosis of anatomic obstruction of the nasal passages. Polyps, severe septal deviation, massive adenoids, or neoplasms may be found.

As mentioned above, examination of the nose begins with notation of the shape of the nasal septum and its contribution to nasal obstruction, but the presence of ulcerations or perforations should be noted. Examination of the nose during uncomplicated allergic rhinitis typically shows edematous, pale, bluish nasal turbinates covered with thin, clear secretions. These inflammatory changes may obstruct the nasal airway and block the ostia draining the sinuses, leading to the complication of sinusitis. A person with allergic rhinitis may have a red mucosa resulting from complications due to the following:
- Viral infections
- Smoking
- Decongestant spray abuse

A pale, edematous mucosa may also be seen in nonallergic rhinitis with eosinophils (NARES). Allergic obstruction of the nose is inherently temporary. When the allergen is gone, the allergic rhinitis improves.

## Laboratory and Skin Tests

The peripheral eosinophil count may be elevated in allergic rhinitis or asthma, but this is nonspecific. A smear of nasal secretions or nasal scraping typically shows polymorphonuclear leukocytes in infectious rhinitis. Eosinophils may predominate in allergic rhinitis, NARES and asthma.

Detection of specific IgE to environmental allergens is usually needed to make a diagnosis of allergic rhinitis. Specific IgE may be detected by immunoassay of a blood sample or by skin tests. Skin testing:
- Has greater sensitivity
- Permits less expensive testing of a larger number of allergens
- Continues to be the method of choice when the skin is suitable for testing

Generalized urticaria or eczema would render the skin unsuitable for testing.

Antihistamines, both $H_1$- and $H_2$-blockers, must be discontinued at least 2 days prior to the skin testing. For antihistamines such as hydroxyzine or astemizole, the patient may need to be off their medication for 1 to 4 weeks to avoid false negative tests. In all patients, control negative (diluent) and control positive (histamine) skin tests should be applied and compared to the allergen skin tests. Both oral and topical corticosteroid therapy do not interfere with immediate hypersensitivity skin testing.

Allergy skin testing materials consist of simple aqueous extracts of proteins from pollens, molds, dust mites and mite fecal pellets, animal danders, and foods. Food extracts are used for diagnosis only. Inhalant extracts are used for skin testing and immunotherapy. A negative intradermal skin test with a normal positive control essentially rules out the presence of specific IgE to the allergen tested. The negative test does not rule out other mechanisms of reaction to an inhaled or ingested substance, but there is no need to consider immunotherapy unless there is a positive skin test. The positive skin test proves the potential for allergic reaction exists but does not prove an allergic mechanism is responsible for the patient's illness.

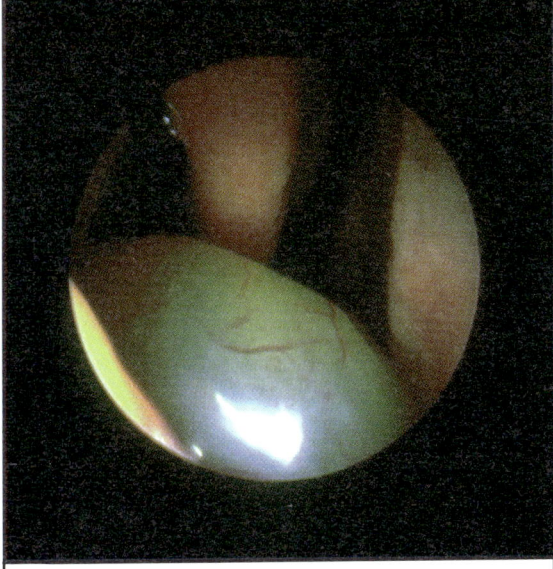

**COLOR PLATE 4.1 — ENDOSCOPIC VIEW OF A NASAL POLYP**

Photo courtesy of Levine HL.

Positive skin tests must be correlated with the clinical history to reach a final diagnosis of allergic rhinitis.

Allergy skin testing usually starts with prick or puncture testing. Comprehensive testing includes individual extracts for locally important trees, grasses and weeds, as well as extracts for cats, dogs, dust mites and molds. A drop of each extract is placed on the skin on the back or arm. A variety of devices are available for puncturing or pricking the skin through the drop. This forces a minute amount of extract into the skin. If specific IgE is present for the antigens tested, wheal and flare reactions develop at the skin test sites

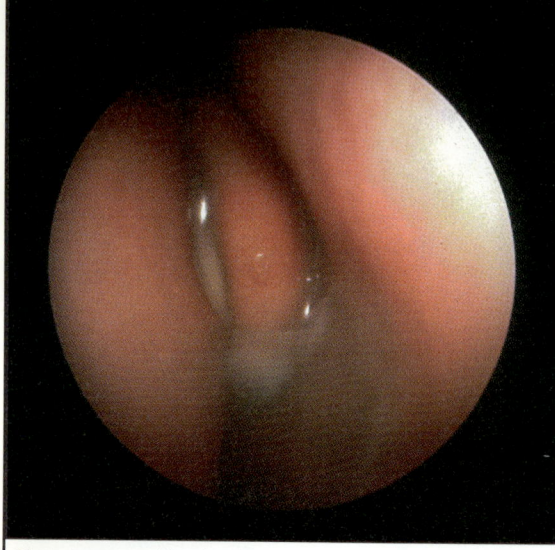

**COLOR PLATE 4.2 — ENDOSCOPIC VIEW OF ACUTE PURULENT SINUSITIS**

Photo courtesy of Levine HL.

within 15 minutes. After the test is read, the excess extract is wiped off the skin.

If prick tests are negative, some physicians go on to intradermal injection of extracts. The extracts used for intradermal testing are at least 25 times more dilute than the extracts used for prick testing. Despite the dilution of the intradermal extract, the intradermal test is more sensitive than the prick test. Some extracts have been standardized for allergenic potency and have their concentration expressed in allergy units (AU) per cc. The higher the number of AU per cc, the more potent the extract.

Some extracts are labeled in the older protein nitrogen units (PNU) per cc. The higher the number of

PNU per cc, the higher the potency of the extract; however, the PNU method is much less accurate than the AU method. Another older system is the weight-by-volume method. A 1:50 ragweed extract consists of the proteins extracted from one gram of ragweed pollen in 50 cc of diluent. The higher the denominator, the more dilute and less potent the extract. Only a few of the many extracts in clinical use have been standardized for allergenic potency. Immunotherapy to a variety of aeroallergens may involve one or more extracts with different units of potency. Preparation of extracts needs to be in the hands of an experienced allergist.

Radioallergosorbent (RAST) or enzyme-linked immunoassays (ELISA) for human IgE to specific allergens are *in vitro* tests that can be run on a serum sample if the skin cannot be used for testing. The main advantage of the *in vitro* assay is safety. The patient is not exposed to the test allergen, and there is no risk of systemic allergic reaction to the allergen. One disadvantage of the *in vitro* test is that a laboratory test needs to be run for each allergen to be tested. The cost of the testing is a direct multiple of the number of tests run. In skin testing, there is little additional cost in testing 20 allergens instead of 10. The results of skin testing are known in 15 minutes, while the results of the *in vitro* test are not known for hours or days. The *in vitro* tests are still less sensitive than skin testing methods in detecting IgE to a specific allergen. For the allergy specialist, skin testing is still the usual method of choice for detection of specific IgE. For both skin testing and *in vitro* testing, positive test results must be considered in light of the clinical history to reach a diagnosis of an allergic illness. Allergy skin tests for ragweed remain positive long after the clinical allergic rhinitis has ceased to recur (Figure 4.1).

**FIGURE 4.1 — OVERLAP IN SERUM IGE LEVELS IN ALLERGIC DISEASE**

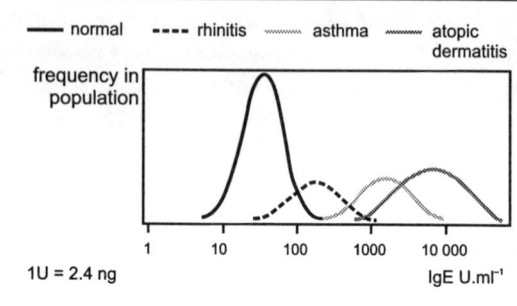

Reproduced from: Holgate ST, Church MK. *Allergy*. London: Mosby; 1993:11.9.

Other laboratory studies such as provocation testing (either nasal or bronchial) with a specific allergen is generally viewed as a research tool.

## Complications of Rhinitis

Complications of chronic inflammation of the nasal passages include:
- Otitis media
- Sinusitis

Otitis is more common in children and sinusitis is more common in adults.

### ■ Otitis Media

Nasal mucosal edema and excess secretions may obstruct the eustachian tube and may result in otitis media. Diagnosis is suggested by:
- Hearing loss
- Ear pain
- Fever
- Delayed speech development in children

Examination may show a retracted tympanic membrane with decreased motion or no motion on pneumatic otoscopy. Tympanometry can document the loss of normal eardrum movement. Audiometry can document a conductive hearing loss. The complication of otitis media may require antibiotic therapy. If middle ear pressure cannot be equalized by medical means, ventilating tubes through the eardrums may be needed.

## ■ Sinusitis

Acute bacterial sinusitis often develops during a severe episode of viral rhinitis. One clinical clue is that after ten days of illness, the nasal symptoms are still not improving and may be getting worse. In the first few days of a viral cold, the symptoms may be as severe as in acute bacterial sinusitis. Computed tomography (CT) scans of the sinuses at this time are likely to be abnormal. However, the patient's illness at this stage is still viral and will not benefit from antibiotics. If the consideration of bacterial sinusitis is deferred until the illness has failed to spontaneously improve in the usual time for a viral cold, the benefit from antimicrobial intervention will be more likely. Allergic rhinitis and viral rhinitis may present with clear rhinorrhea, nasal congestion, and sneezing. Allergic rhinitis usually does not progress to the thick yellow discharge of viral or bacterial infection. Ocular itching and watering are usually more prominent in allergic rhinitis. For many patients with allergic rhinitis, exposure to aeroallergens is intermittent. This results in natural periods of time without symptoms. These patients usually do not develop sinusitis. When there is constant exposure to allergens, nasal congestion may be persistent enough to lead to sinusitis.

Chronic sinusitis frequently involves eosinophilic inflammation of the sinus mucosa similar to the eosinophilic inflammation in the asthmatic airway. Some, but not all of these patients have inhalant allergies.

Nasal polyps are found in over 25% of cases with opacification of or air fluid levels in the frontal, maxillary or sphenoid sinuses. Each sinus has a small opening or ostium through which mucus normally vacates the sinus propelled by the dilated epithelium. The maxillary, sphenoidal and frontal sinuses are large, paired, bony chambers, whereas the ethmoid sinuses consist of a labyrinth of small bony cells (see Figure 4.2).

Obstruction of the ostium of any of these cells leads to accumulation of secretions in the sinus cavity

**FIGURE 4.2 — NORMAL OSTIOMEATAL COMPLEX (CORONAL VIEW)**

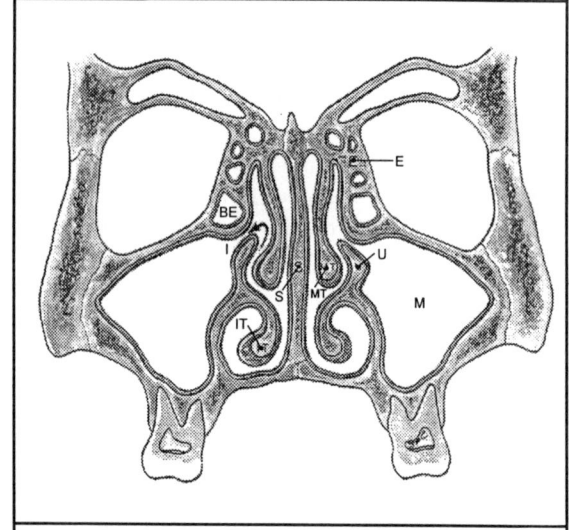

BE: bulla ethmoidalis; I: maxillary sinus infundibulum; U: uncinate process; IT: inferior turbinate; S: nasal septum; MT: middle turbinate; E: ethmoids; Curved arrow: hiatus semilunare.

Levine HL, May M, (eds). *Endoscopic Sinus Surgery*. New York: Thieme; 1993:247.

with the potential for eventual bacterial sinusitis. The maxillary sinuses, the frontal sinuses, and the anterior ethmoid air cells all drain into the middle meatus beneath the middle turbinate. The normal middle meatus is only a few millimeters wide. Mucosal inflammation easily obstructs sinus outflow (see Figure 4.3). If the obstruction persists long enough, infection is likely.

Infection results in more mucosal inflammation, leading to chronic sinusitis. The maxillary cavities are the sinuses most frequently involved in sinusitis. Under normal conditions, the ciliated mucosal cells move a blanket of mucus upward to the apex of the

**FIGURE 4.3 — OSTIOMEATAL COMPLEX OBSTRUCTION AND SECONDARY SINUSITIS (CORONAL VIEW)**

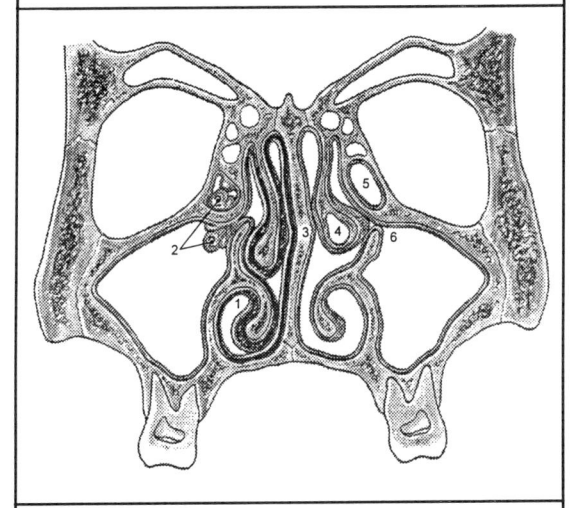

1) inflammatory (obstructive) changes; 2) polyps (maxillary and ethmoid sinuses); 3) septal deviation; 4) paradoxical middle turbinate and concha bullosa; 5) large bulla ethmoidalis; 6) ostiomeatal complex stenosis.

maxillary sinus. The mucus must move up over the uncinate process and down under the middle turbinate to reach the nasal passage. This narrow path is easily obstructed by swollen mucosa. The ethmoid air cells are the second most commonly involved sinuses in chronic sinusitis. The frontal and sphenoid sinuses are far less frequently involved despite the common complaint of a frontal "sinus headache."

Sinus obstruction may be secondary to a number of conditions including:
- Nasal allergy
- Respiratory infection
- Overuse of topical decongestants
- Deviated nasal septum
- Nasal polyps (frequent cause of pansinusitis)
- Tumors
- Foreign bodies
- Cystic fibrosis

Sinusitis can be broadly classified as acute or chronic. Acute sinusitis is an infectious process of the paranasal sinuses, which lasts from 1 day to 3 weeks and is characterized by:
- Pain or tenderness over the maxillary sinuses
- Upper molar toothache
- Purulent nasal drainage
- Nasal obstruction

Acute sinusitis often occurs following a viral upper respiratory tract infection. The typical bacterial pathogens in acute sinusitis include:
- *S. pneunoniae*
- *H. influenza*
- *M. catarrhalis*

Untreated, acute sinusitis may progress to meningitis or epidural abscess.

Chronic sinusitis is an inflammatory process of the paranasal sinuses lasting 3 months or more. Symptoms of chronic sinusitis may include:
- Rhinorrhea
- Thick postnasal drainage
- Facial pain
- Chronic headaches
- Halitosis
- Chronic nasal obstruction
- Cough
- Treatment-resistant asthma

Pathogens in chronic sinusitis may include the pathogens of acute sinusitis as well as anaerobic pathogens such as:
- *Peptostreptococcus*
- *Corynebacterium*
- *Bacteroides* species

## ■ Diagnosing Sinusitis

Clinical history including yellow or green nasal drainage and facial pressure or pain raises the diagnostic possibility of sinusitis, but no one symptom has both high sensitivity and specificity. Nasal speculum examination is limited to evaluation of the anterior portion of the nasal passages. Rhinoscopy may firmly establish a diagnosis of sinusitis if purulent discharge is observed streaming from beneath the middle or superior turbinate (Figures 4.4, Color Plates 4.1 and 4.2 [see pages 33 and 34]). However, in many cases, firm proof of sinusitis may only be obtained radiographically. Plain x-rays may provide adequate information to identify sinusitis in the maxillary or frontal sinuses, but plain films are inadequate to evaluate the ethmoid air cells. In all cases, CT images provide far more details of the sinus anatomy than plain films (Figures 4.5 through 4.14). Several studies have demonstrated

**FIGURE 4.4 — ENDOSCOPIC VIEW OF RIGHT UNCINATE PROCESS**

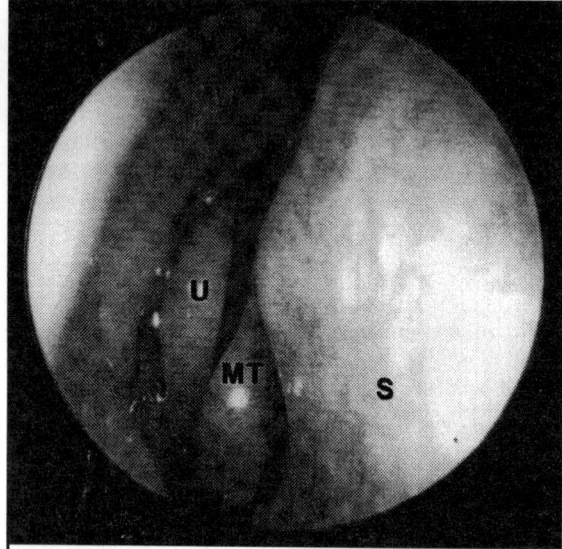

U: uncinate; MT: middle turbinate; S: septum.

Reproduced from: Levine HL, May M (eds). *Endoscopic Sinus Surgery*. New York: Thieme; 1993:83.

that 4 to 6 cuts in either the coronal or axial plane are sufficient to evaluate for sinusitis. If sinus surgery is to be performed, more detailed coronal cuts are needed. Radiographic images reveal mucosal and bony abnormalities. They do not reveal the presence or absence of bacteria. However, air fluid levels and opacified sinus cavities correlate well with positive sinus cultures. The severity and nature of symptoms in the presence of mucosal abnormality on the CT scan determines the need for medical or surgical intervention.

An isolated episode of suspected sinusitis may be treated with antibiotics without proof by CT scan. If acute sinusitis is recurring frequently or a diagnosis of

**FIGURE 4.5 — SIMPLE CT OF NORMAL SINUSES (AXIAL VIEWS)**

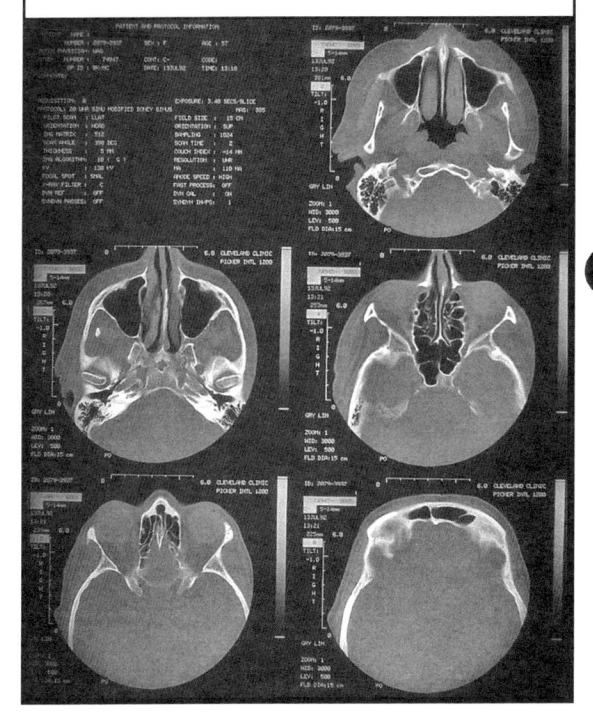

chronic sinusitis is being made, confirmation by limited CT scan is recommended. Current treatment of chronic sinusitis includes antibiotics for a minimum of 3 weeks. The failure of a 10-day course of antibiotics is identified by the return of symptoms within a few days of discontinuation of the antibiotic. The antibiotic used must be appropriate for beta lactamase-producing organisms. If symptoms persist despite appropriate antibiotics for 3 weeks or more, rhinoscopy should be performed to identify anatomic impairment to sinus drainage. Nasal polyps are the most common anatomic factor contributing to the persistence or re-

**FIGURE 4.6 — SIMPLE CT OF SINUSES (DEVIATED SEPTUM, NO SINUSITIS [CORONAL VIEW])**

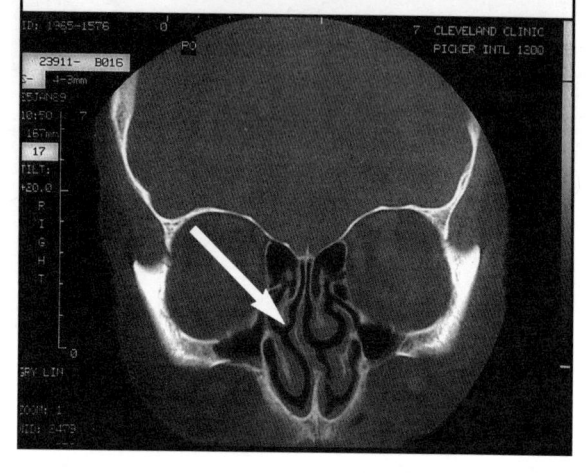

currence of chronic sinusitis. Unfortunately, the surgical removal of nasal polyps can only be considered a temporary measure. The natural history of nasal polyps is recurrence. Yet, if the nasal passages are completely blocked, or if infection in the sinuses is unresponsive to nasal steroids and antibiotics, surgical removal of polyps must be done. Even in the absence of polyps, persisting sinusitis may need surgical improvement of drainage to heal. Fortunately, sinus surgery now is usually performed endoscopically with much less trauma to the patient.

If drainage is not blocked, yet infection is recurrent, evaluation of the humoral immune system should be considered. IgA deficiency is the most common humoral deficiency in the general population; however, not all patients with IgA deficiency will have frequent infections. The IgA deficient patients who also have an IgG subclass deficiency seem more prone to

**FIGURE 4.7 — SIMPLE CT OF SINUSES SHOWING EXTENSIVE BILATERAL SINUSITIS (AXIAL VIEWS)**

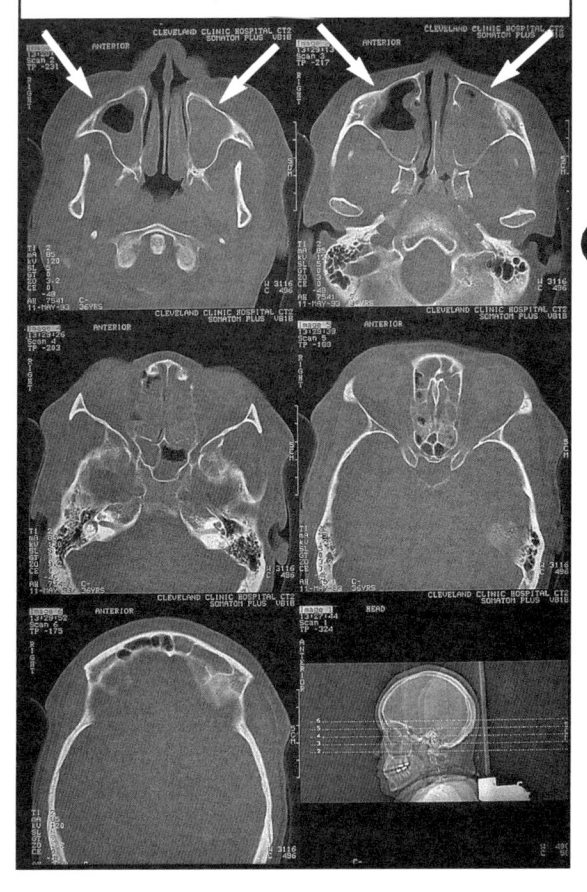

infection. The humoral evaluation is not limited to measurement of the levels of IgG, IgA, IgM and the IgG subclasses. Part of the evaluation of the functional status of the humoral immune system includes measurement of antibodies to specific antigens such as tetanus toxoid and pneumococcal antigens. Some

**FIGURE 4.8 — SIMPLE CT DEMONSTRATES THAT THE LEFT MAXILLARY SINUS IS SMALLER, WITHOUT SINUSITIS (AXIAL VIEW)**

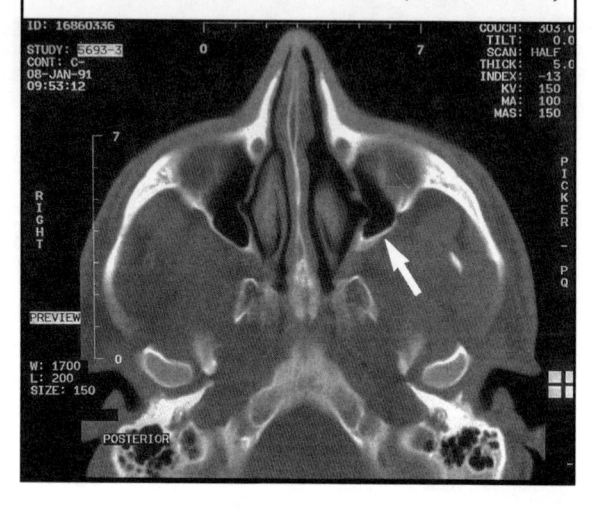

patients fail to make specific antibodies despite normal antibodies class and subclass levels. Tetanus and pneumococcal antibody levels can be measured before and after immunization. Demonstration of a 4-fold rise in specific antibody in 1 month after immunization confirms immune competence. A very small percentage of patients with chronic sinusitis will be found to have a humoral immune deficiency requiring intravenous gammaglobulin treatment in addition to antibiotics. Patients with IgA deficiency alone are not candidates for intravenous gammaglobulin. In fact, they are at risk for allergic reaction if given intravenous gammaglobulin. Common variable hypogammaglobulinemia is associated with chronic sinusitis, otitis media in adults, and recurrent pneumonia and is appropriately treated with monthly intravenous gammaglobulin.

**FIGURE 4.9 — PLAIN X-RAY FALSELY SHOWING OPACIFICATION OF LEFT MAXILLARY SINUS**

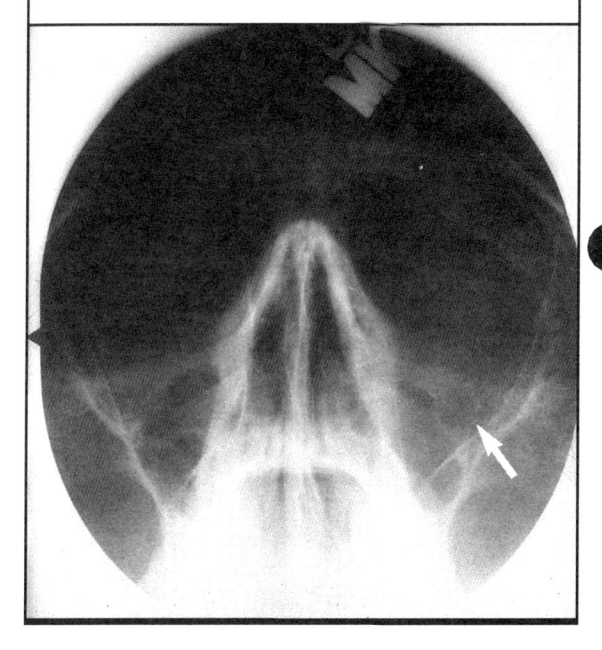

Establishment of normal mucus drainage from the sinuses is an integral part of healing sinusitis. Oral decongestants, decongestant nasal sprays (for a few days), saline nasal sprays, and steroid nasal sprays may help restore sinus drainage. Oral antihistamines and steroid nasal sprays are also used when the underlying illness is allergic rhinitis. Steroid nasal sprays are especially important when nasal polyps have caused the sinusitis.

If a complication of sinusitis develops, such as penetration of infection into the cranium or the orbit, the case is a surgical and medical emergency. Surgical intervention is also needed if drainage of the sinuses cannot be achieved medically.

**FIGURE 4.10 — SIMPLE CT DEMONSTRATES A LARGE LEFT MAXILLARY POLYP WITHOUT EVIDENCE OF SINUSITIS (AXIAL VIEWS)**

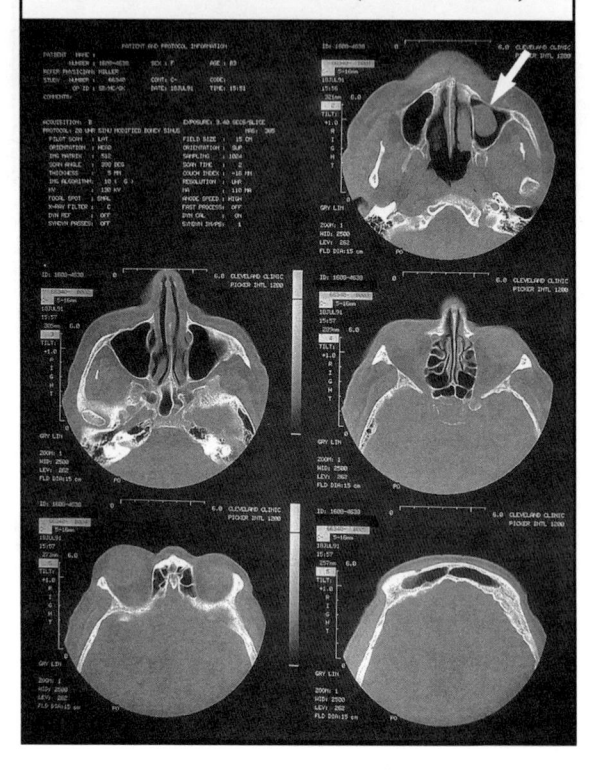

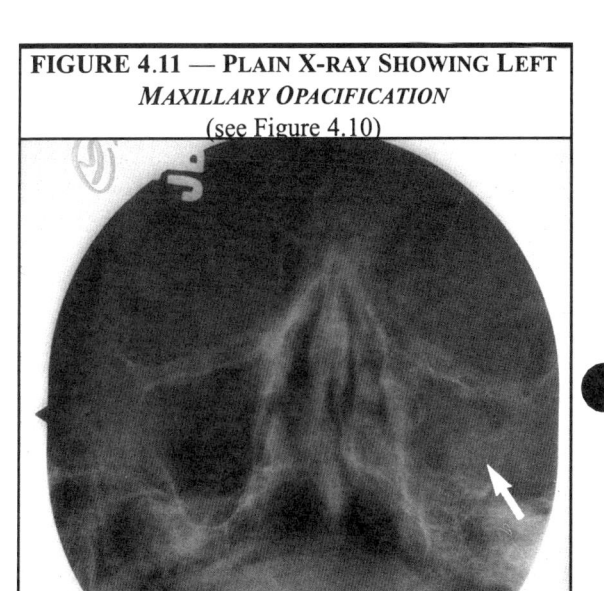

**FIGURE 4.11 — PLAIN X-RAY SHOWING LEFT *MAXILLARY OPACIFICATION*** 
(see Figure 4.10)

**FIGURE 4.12 — PLAIN X-RAY SHOWING AIR FLUID LEVEL IN THE LEFT MAXILLARY SINUS**

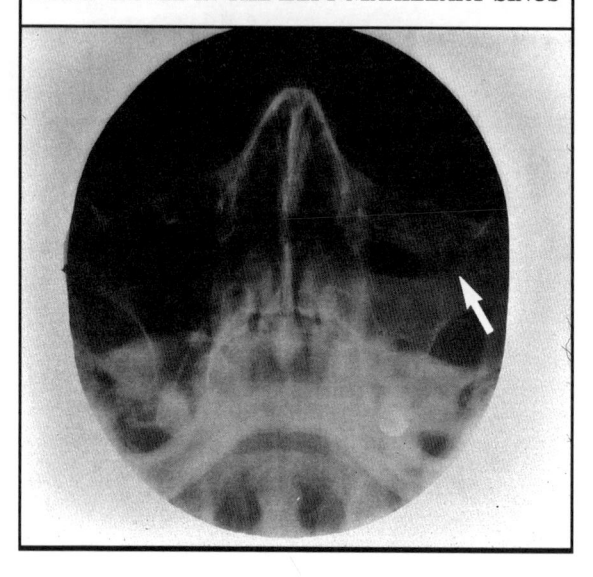

**FIGURE 4.13 — SIMPLE CT DEMONSTRATES A LARGE BONY SPUR OF THE SEPTUM (AXIAL VIEWS)**

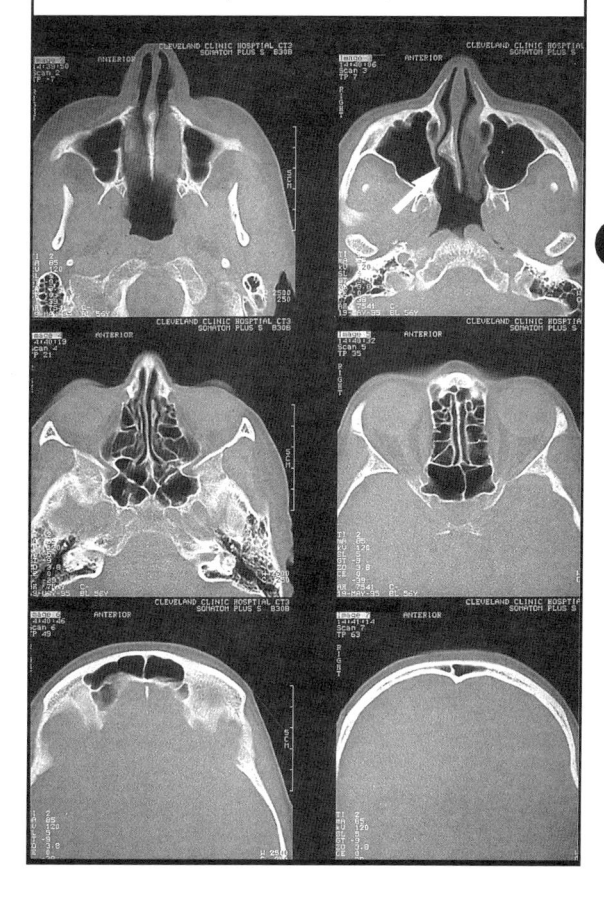

**FIGURE 4.14 — CT SHOWS A LARGE NEUROBLASTOMA ENCROACHING INTO THE SEPTUM (CORONAL VIEW)**

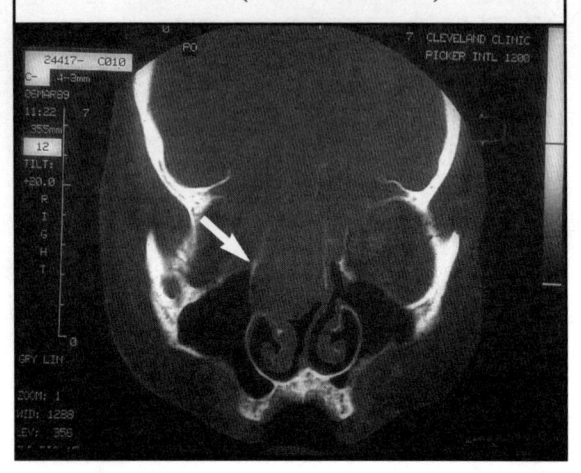

# PART 3

# THERAPY FOR RHINITIS

# 5 Nonpharmacological Therapy

The general goals of therapy for chronic rhinitis syndrome include:
- Restoration of nasal patency
- Control of nasal secretions
- Treatment of complications such as bacterial infection

There are 3 specific approaches for management:
- Avoidance of the responsible allergens
- Pharmacotherapy (see Chapter 6):
  - Antihistamines
  - Decongestants
  - Intranasal corticosteroids
  - Cromolyn sodium
  - Anticholinergics
  - Ocular therapy
- Immunotherapy by subcutaneous injection of increasing quantities of allergen (in selected patients) (see Chapter 7)

## Avoidance of Responsible Allergens

Allergy skin testing is essential for management of chronic rhinitis if immunotherapy is being considered. The results of skin tests are helpful in establishment of a diagnosis and in treatment, even when immunotherapy is not being considered. The skin test results guide recommendations concerning any environmental control that may be needed. In seasonal rhinitis, the skin tests usually confirm pollen sensitivity. Outdoor pollen cannot be avoided, but the indoor pollen count can be greatly reduced by use of air conditioning, thus permitting the windows to be closed during pollen season. Air conditioning should also be used in the car during pollen season. Patients with pollen or mold allergy should not mow the grass or rake leaves. In year-round, chronic rhinitis, dust mite allergens and animal dander allergens may be contributing factors. Dust mite control measures (Table 5.1) can reduce respiratory symptoms; but some steps, such as removing carpeting, are fairly drastic and should only be recommended for those with proven mite sensitivity. Advice regarding pets can only be given after specific sensitivity has been tested. Avoidance of smoke is a necessary part of chronic rhinitis management, even though smoke is an irritant rather than a true allergen.

### TABLE 5.1 — HOUSE-DUST MITE CONTROL MEASURES

**Essential**:
- Encase the mattress in an airtight cover
- Either encase the pillow or wash it weekly
- Wash the bedding in water of 130° F weekly
- Avoid sleeping or lying on upholstered furniture
- Remove carpets that are laid on concrete

**Desirable**:
- Reduce indoor humidity to less than 50%
- Remove carpets from the bedroom
- Use chemical agents to kill mites or to alter the mite antigens in the house

Reproduced from: National Asthma Education Program: expert panel report. *Guidelines for the Diagnosis and Management of Asthma.* Bethesda, MD: National Institutes of Health; 1991:66.

# 6 Pharmacological Therapy

Pharmacological agents available for the treatment of rhinitis include:
- Antihistamines
- Decongestants
- Intranasal corticosteroids
- Cromolyn sodium
- Anticholinergics
- Ocular therapy

(Also see Table 6.1.)

## Antihistamines

Histamine remains an important mediator of symptoms in allergic rhinitis and conjunctivitis. Histamine-receptor antagonists are widely prescribed for symptomatic management of allergic rhinitis. These agents are very effective in controlling nasal itching, rhinorrhea, and sneezing; but they are less effective in controlling nasal congestion (see Table 6.2). Antihistamines work by preventing the binding of histamine in the target tissue. They do not reverse any action already taken by histamine. Based on this observation, antihistamines work best when taken daily during a period of allergen exposure. In addition to competitively blocking the binding of histamine by $H_1$-receptors, some of the agents in this class also block the release of histamine and perhaps other mediators from mast cells. In addition, recent work suggests that antihistamines may also block the influx of eosinophils following allergen challenge.

## TABLE 6.1 — CURRENTLY AVAILABLE PHARMACOLOGIC AGENTS FOR TREATMENT OF RHINITIS

**Antihistamines** (Table 6.3)
- First generation
- Second generation

**Inhaled Sympathomimetics** (Table 6.4)

- *Short-acting*
  - Epinephrine
  - Naphazoline
  - Phenylephrine
  - Tetrahydrozoline
- *Long-acting*
  - Oxymetazoline
  - Xylometazoline

**Oral Sympathomimetics** (Table 6.4)

- Phenylpropanolamine
- Pseudoephedrine

**Steroid Nasal Inhalers** (Table 6.5)

- Beclomethasone dipropionate
- Budesonide
- Dexamethasone sodium phosphate
- Flunisolide
- Fluticasone
- Triamcinolone acetonide

**Cromoglycates** (Table 6.7)

- Cromolyn sodium solution

**Anticholinergics** (Table 6.7)

- Ipratropium bromide

**Hybrid Nasal Sprays** (Table 6.4)

### TABLE 6.2 — RELATIVE EFFICACY OF DRUGS IN TREATMENT OF ALLERGIC RHINITIS

| | Symptoms | | |
|---|---|---|---|
| Drug | Sneezing | Congestion | Secretions |
| Antihistamine | ++ | − | + |
| Decongestant | − | ++ | − |
| Nasal steroid | ++ | ++ | ++ |
| Cromolyn sodium | + | + | + |
| Anticholinergic | − | − | ++ |

Antihistamines can be broadly classified as:
- First generation (sedating)
  - Brompheniramine
  - Chlorpheniramine
  - Hydroxyzine
- Second generation (non- or mildly-sedating):
  - Astemizole
  - Cetirizine
  - Loratadine
  - Terfenadine

See Table 6.3 for classification of $H_1$-receptor antagonists.

Numerous placebo-controlled, prospective studies have clearly shown that both first and second generation antihistamines are effective in controlling the symptoms of allergic rhinitis except congestion. Sedative and anticholinergic effects of first generation antihistamines account for most of the adverse side effects. Decreased alertness may be demonstrable even if patients deny sedation.

There are some differences in the duration of action in both first and second generation antihistamines.

## TABLE 6.3 — AVAILABLE $H_1$-ANTIHISTAMINES

| Class/Generic Name | Trade Name (Manufacturer) | Dosage (Adult) | Dosage (Children 12 years & under) |
|---|---|---|---|
| **FIRST GENERATION ANTIHISTAMINES** ||||
| *Alkylamines* <br> Brompheniramine maleate | Dimetane* (A.H. Robins) | 4 mg, 3-4 times/d | 0.4 mg/kg, in 3-4 divided doses/d |
| Chlorpheniramine maleate | Chlor-trimeton* (Schering) | 4 mg, 3-4 times/d | < 2 y, 1.25 mg, 2-3 times daily; 0.4 mg/kg in 3-4 divided doses/d |
| *Ethanolamine* <br> Diphenhydramine hydrochloride | Benadryl* (Parke-Davis) | 25-50 mg, 3-4 times/d | 5 mg/kg, in 3-4 divided doses/d |
| *Ethylenediamines* <br> Tripelennamine hydrochloride | PBZ Pyribenzamine* (Geigy) | 25-30 mg, 3-4 times/d | 5 mg/kg, in 3-4 divided doses/d |
| *Phenothiazines* <br> Promethazine hydrochloride | Phenergan† (Wyeth-Ayerst) | 12.5-25 mg, 2-3 times/d | 1 mg/kg per hour, divided into doses at bedtime and quarter doses in daytime |

| | | | |
|---|---|---|---|
| *Piperazines* | | | |
| Azatadine maleate | Optimine† (Schering) | 1-2 mg, 2 times/d | No recommendation |
| Hydroxyzine hydrochloride | Atarax† (Roerig/Pfizer) | 10-50 mg, 3-4 times/d | 2 mg/kg, in 4 divided doses/d |
| | Vistaril† (Roerig/Pfizer) | 10-50 mg, 3-4 times/d | 2 mg/kg, in 4 divided doses/d |
| *Miscellaneous* | | | |
| Clemastine fumarate | Tavist 1*, Tavist D*, Tavist† (Sandoz) | 1.34 mg, 2.68 mg, 2 times/d | No recommendation |
| Cyproheptadine hydrochloride | Periactin* (Merck, Sharp & Dohme) | 4 mg, 3-4 times/d | 0.25 mg/kg, in 3-4 divided doses/d |
| **SECOND GENERATION (NON-SEDATING OR MILDLY SEDATING) ANTIHISTAMINES** | | | |
| Astemizole | Hismanal† (Janssen) | 10 mg/d | No recommendation |
| Cetirizine | Zyrtec† (Pfizer) | 10 mg/d | 5-10 mg/d |
| Loratadine | Claritin† (Schering) | 10 mg/d | 5-10 mg/d |
| Terfenadine | Seldane† (Marion Merrell Dow) | 60 mg, 2 times/d | No recommendation |
| Fexofenadine‡ | Allegra† (Hoechst-Marion Roussel) | 60 mg, 2 times/d | No recommendation |

\* Over-the-counter preparation    † Prescription only    ‡ Investigational in United States

Modified with permission from: Kaliner M, Lemanske R. Rhinitis and Asthma. *JAMA*.1992;268:2814.

Specifically, in the first generation, durations of action are as follows:
- Brompheniramine—3 to 9 hours
- Chlorpheniramine—24 hours
- Hydroxyzine—36 hours

Among the second generation antihistamines, durations of action are as follows:
- Terfenadine—12 to 24 hours
- Loratadine and cetirizine—24 hours
- Astemizole—very long acting, up to several weeks

Much of this data was obtained by an experimental model involving cutaneous wheal suppression by the oral administration of these agents. Using this model, there appear to be some differences in relative potency of these agents with the following ranking from the most potent to least potent:
- Cetirizine
- Terfenadine
- Loratadine
- Astemizole
- Chlorpheniramine
- Placebo

A common and troublesome side effect of the first generation antihistamines is sedation. Since these agents are nonprotein bound, they penetrate the central nervous system and bind to central $H_1$-receptors and, hence, produce sedation. A number of studies suggest that the incidence of sedation may be 20% in patients using the older antihistamines, although the incidence of more subtle impaired performance may be substantially higher. At the recommended doses, the second generation antihistamines do not appear to have significant sedation or performance impairment compared to placebo. However, loratadine at doses of

40 mg and cetirizine at 20 mg (both above the recommended doses for these agents) may cause sedation.

The first generation antihistamines are also more likely to cause anticholinergic effects. This could result in urinary retention, especially in the elderly. The incidence of this side effect is much less for the second generation antihistamines. Appetite stimulation has been occasionally noted with astemizole.

Terfenadine and astemizole have been associated with cardiac arrhythmias, with rare fatalities. There are over 25 cases of torsade de pointes in the Food and Drug Administration (FDA) database. The arrhythmias have mostly occurred with:
- Excessive doses of these agents
- Concomitant administration of a variety of drugs including:
  - Azoles (chlotrimazole, fluconazole, itraconazole, ketoconazole, miconazole)
  - Macrolides (clarithromycin, erythromycin, troleandomycin)
  - Others (quinine)
- Underlying liver disease

Torsade de pointes is a clinical syndrome in which polymorphic ventricular tachycardia occurs in the setting of antecedent prolongation of the Q-T interval. A number of studies strongly suggest that a quinidine-like effect, or prolongation of the Q-T interval by delay of repolarization, is the likely mechanism involved in antihistamine-related torsade de pointes. Azoles, macrolides and underlying liver disease have the effect of increasing the parent drug levels of both terfenadine and astemizole. There have been no reports to date of torsade de pointes in association with either loratadine or cetirizine.

Some authors have expressed concern over the use of terfenadine and astemizole in a number of other settings where the Q-T interval may be prolonged, such as:

- Congenital Q-T prolongation
- Concomitant use of other antiarrhythmics:
  - Class IA (quinidine, procainamide, disopyramide)
  - Class III (amiodarone, sotalol)
- Electrolyte abnormalities
  - Hypomagnesemia
  - Hypokalemia

Early reports in the 1970s suggested that antihistamines may be relatively contraindicated in patients with co-existent allergic rhinitis and bronchial asthma. This was based on the thought that excessive drying of the respiratory tract may exacerbate bronchospasm. However, subsequent experience in the last 10 to 15 years suggests that antihistamines are quite effective and safe for the symptomatic treatment of allergic rhinitis, even in patients with bronchial asthma. In fact, there is preliminary data that cetirizine may be useful in inhibiting histamine-mediated smooth muscle contraction (bronchospasm) associated with exercise-mediated or allergen-mediated asthma.

## Decongestants

Nasal congestion is one of the most common complaints from patients with chronic rhinitis. Antihistamines do not adequately relieve this symptom for many people and additional intervention is needed. If obstruction is intermittent and cannot be attributed to the shape of nasal bone and cartilage, thickness of the soft tissues of the nose need to be reduced. The thickness of the soft tissues is influenced by edema of the mucosa and by the engorgement of the venous sinusoids. Decongestant nasal sprays reduce the amount of blood in the venous sinusoids, thereby reducing the volume of space occupied by the turbinates. Phenylephrine, oxymetazoline, xylometazoline and naphazoline are alpha-agonists (Table 6.4). They are potent vasoconstrictors. When used for more than 5 to 7 consecutive days, rebound congestion develops upon withdrawal of the drug. Prolonged use leads to rhinitis medicamentosa. The topical decongestants may be used for acute viral rhinitis but not for allergic rhinitis, which has an expected duration of weeks or months.

The oral decongestants pseudoephedrine and phenylpropanolamine are commonly combined with antihistamines to improve relief from nasal congestion. The principal side effects of oral decongestants are as follows:

- Nervousness
- Insomnia
- Irritability
- Headache
- Palpitations
- Tachycardia

Oral decongestants may interfere with urinary flow in males and are contraindicated in patients with:

- Hypertension
- Severe coronary artery disease
- Monoamine oxidase inhibitor (MAOI) therapy

Prolonged use of oral decongestants on a daily basis may lead to withdrawal symptoms of headache and fatigue when the drug is stopped.

## Intranasal Corticosteroids

The pharmacologic effect of corticosteroids requires hours to take effect due to the multiple intracellular and intranuclear events necessary to produce post transcriptional proteins. These proteins inhibit multiple steps in the inflammatory process. As summarized by Meltzer, they:

- Cause vasoconstriction

## TABLE 6.4 — DECONGESTANTS*

| Generic Name | Trade Name (Manufacturer) | Delivery Device | Dosage (Adults) |
|---|---|---|---|
| **INHALED SYMPATHOMIMETICS — *Short-Acting*** ||||
| Ephedrine hydrochloride | Efedron Gel (Hyrex) | Nasal jelly | Small amount each nostril q 4 h |
| Naphazoline hydrochloride | Privine (CIBA Consumer) | Drops | 1-2 drops each nostril q 3-4 h prn |
| | | Sprays | 1-2 sprays each nostril q 3-4 h prn |
| Phenylephrine | Duration (Schering-Plough) | Spray (mild strength) | 1-2 sprays each nostril q 4 h prn |
| | | Spray (regular strength) | 1-2 sprays each nostril q 4 h prn |
| hydrochloride | Neo-Synephrine (Sanofi Winthrop) | Drop (mild strength) | 1-2 drops each nostril q 4 h prn |
| | | Spray (mild strength) | 1-2 sprays each nostril q 4 h prn |
| | | Drop (regular strength) | 1-2 drops each nostril q 4 h prn |
| | | Spray (regular strength) | 1-2 sprays each nostril q 4 h prn |
| | Nostril (CIBA Consumer) | Spray (mild strength) | 1-2 sprays each nostril q 4 h prn |
| | | Spray (regular strength) | 1-2 sprays each nostril q 4 h prn |
| | Vicks – Sinex (Proctor and Gamble) | Spray | 1-2 sprays each nostril q 4 h prn |

| Tetrahydrozoline hydrochloride | Tyzine (Kenwood) | Solution | 2-4 drops each nostril q 4-6 h prn |
|---|---|---|---|
| **INHALED SYMPATHOMIMETICS — *Long-Acting*** | | | |
| Oxymetazoline hydrochloride | Afrin (Schering-Plough) | Spray | 2-4 sprays each nostril bid |
| | Decongest (Truxton) | Spray | 2-4 sprays each nostril bid |
| | Dristan Long-Lasting (Whitehall) | Spray | 2-4 sprays each nostril bid |
| | Neo-Synephrine 12-Hour (Sterling Health) | Spray | 2-4 sprays each nostril bid |
| | Neo-Synephrine Maximum Strength (Sterling Health) | Spray | 2-4 sprays each nostril bid |
| | Nostrilla (CIBA Consumer) | Drops | 2-4 drops each nostril bid |
| | | Spray | 2-4 sprays each nostril bid |
| Xylometazoline hydrochloride | Otrixin (CIBA Consumer) | Drops | 2-3 drops each nostril q 8-10 h |
| | | Spray | 1-2 sprays each nostril q 8-10 h |
| | Sinex Long-Acting (P&G, Richardson VI) | Spray | 1-2 sprays each nostril q 8-10 h |

| Generic Name | Trade Name (Manufacturer) | Delivery Device | Dosage (Adults) |
|---|---|---|---|
| **ORAL SYMPATHOMIMETICS** | | | |
| Pseudoephedrine hydrochloride | Novafed (Marion Merrell Dow) | Capsule | 120 mg (1 capsule) po q 12 h |
| | Pseudogest (Major) | Syrup | 60 mg (2 tsps) po q 4 h |
| | | Tablet | 60 mg po q 4 h |
| | Sudafed (Burroughs Wellcome) | Tablet | 60 mg po q 4 h |
| | Sudafed 12 Hr. (Burroughs Wellcome) | Tablet | 120 mg po q 12 h |
| **HYBRID INTRANASAL SPRAYS** | | | |
| Phenylephrine HCL/ naphazoline HCL/ pyrilamine maleate | 4-Way Fast-Acting (Bristol-Myers) | Nasal spray metered pump | 1-2 sprays each nostril q 3-4 h |
| Phenylephrine HCL/ pheniramine maleate | Dristal Nasal (Whitehall) | Nasal spray | 1-2 sprays each nostril q 3-4 h |
| Phenylephine HCL/ pyrilamine maleate | MYCl Spray (Misemer) | Nasal spray | 1-2 sprays each nostril q 3-4 h |

\* Over-the-counter preparations

- Decrease glandular response to cholinergic stimulation
- Interfere with arachidonic acid metabolism
- Reduce mediator release
- Decrease production of cytokines from $T_{H2}$ lymphocytes
- Inhibit influx of eosinophils to the nasal epithelium

Topical nasal steroid sprays are the most potent medications available for the treatment of allergic rhinitis. Available nasal steroid sprays include (Table 6.5):
- Beclomethasone
- Budesonide
- Dexamethasone
- Flunisolide
- Fluticasone
- Triamcinolone acetonide

Budesonide and fluticasone are the most topically potent, using a vasoconstrictor index of potency (Table 6.6). Within the dosage range recommended by the manufacturers, there is minimal evidence for systemic effect of these topical sprays because of low systemic absorption and first pass metabolism through the liver. The older dexamethasone spray does have significant suppressive effect on adrenal function. Nasal steroid sprays effectively reduce nasal mucosal congestion, sneezing, and rhinorrhea; but they need to be combined with antihistamine to effectively control eye symptoms. Once or twice daily dosing is sufficient for the steroid sprays. Both aqueous pump spray and pressurized aerosol forms are available. Studies of the safety of long-term nasal steroid use do not reveal any nasal candidiasis or evidence of nasal mucosal damage in 48 weeks. Bleeding from the anterior nasal septum has been reported with nasal steroid use. This

## TABLE 6.5 — STEROID NASAL INHALERS

| Class/Generic Name | Trade Name (Manufacturer) | Delivery Device | Dosage (Adults) |
|---|---|---|---|
| Beclomethasone dipropionate | Beconase (Allen/Hanburys) | Aerosol inhaler | 1 spray each nostril bid-qid (42 mcg/spray) |
| | Beconase AQ (Allen/Hanburys) | Pump spray | 1-2 sprays each nostril bid (42 mcg/spray) |
| | Vancenase (Schering) | Aerosol inhaler | 1 spray each nostril bid-qid (42 mcg/spray) |
| | Vancenase AQ (Schering) | Pump spray | 1-2 sprays each nostril bid (42 mcg/spray) |
| Budesonide | Rhinocort (Astra) | Aerosol inhaler | 2-4 sprays each nostril qd (32 mcg/spray) |
| Dexamethasone sodium phosphate | Dexacort (Adams) | Aerosol inhaler | 2 sprays each nostril bid-tid; max dose=12 sprays/d (100 mcg/spray) |
| Flunisolide | Nasalide (Syntex) | Pump spray | 2 sprays each nostril bid; max dose=8 sprays/d (25 mcg/spray) |
| | Nasarel (Roche) | Pump spray | 1-2 sprays each nostril bid; max dose = 8 sprays/d (25 mcg/spray) |
| Fluticasone propionate | Flonase (Glaxo, Allen/Hanburys) | Pump spray | 1-2 sprays each nostril qd (50 mcg/spray) |
| Triamcinolone acetonide | Nasacort (Rhone Poulenc Rorer) | Aerosol inhaler | 2-4 sprays each nostril qd (55 mcg/spray) |

| TABLE 6.6 — RELATIVE TOPICAL VASOCONSTRICTOR POTENCY ||
|---|---|
| Drug | Activity |
| Hydrocortisone | 1 |
| Triamcinolone | 1,000 |
| Flunisolide | 3,000 |
| Beclomethasone | 5,000 |
| Budesonide | 10,000 |
| Fluticasone | 10,000 |

Modified from Melter EO. An overview of current pharmacotherapy in perennial rhinitis. *J Allergy Clin Immunol*. 1995; 95:1097-1110; and Siegel SC. Topical intranasal corticosteroid therapy in rhinitis. *J Allergy Clin Immunol*. 1988;81:984-991.

problem may be minimized by directing the spray away from the septum and by using lower velocity sprays.

## Cromolyn Sodium

Cromolyn sodium is also effective for symptomatic control of both seasonal and perennial allergic rhinitis. Cromolyn sodium is able to prevent both the acute phase and late phase reactions to allergen. In general, cromolyn sodium should be administered prophylactically before exposure. Cromolyn sodium appears to be effective, but less potent than nasal corticosteroids. The safety profile of cromolyn sodium is excellent (Table 6.7).

## Anticholinergics

Anticholinergics are known to be drying agents. There is currently only one topical anticholinergic agent available — ipratropium bromide nasal spray.

## TABLE 6.7 — MISCELLANEOUS AGENTS FOR RHINITIS

| Generic Name | Trade Name (Manufacturer) | Delivery Device | Dosage (Adults) |
|---|---|---|---|
| Cromolyn solution | Nasalcrom (Fisons) | Solution (metered inhaler) | 1 spray each nostril tid-qid up to 6/d |
| Ipratropium bromide | Atrovent Nasal Spray (Boehringer Ingelheim) | Nasal spray (0.03%, 0.06%) | 2 sprays each nostril tid-qid |
| Azelastine* | Astelin (Carter-Wallace) | Nasal spray | — |

* Investigational in the United States

Rhinorrhea is predominantly cholinergically mediated. Ipratropium blocks the hypersecretory effects of the cholinergic neurotransmitter acetylcholine by competing with it for binding sites on the cell.

Ipratropium nasal spray is effective in reducing rhinorrhea associated with allergic and nonallergic rhinitis and the common cold. It is equally effective in all three conditions. When compared with nasal saline, which can itself be beneficial in treatment of rhinitis, ipratropium therapy resulted in a 30% reduction in rhinorrhea. There was less significant reduction in postnasal drip, congestion and sneezing. Preliminary data suggests that ipratropium produces additional control of rhinorrhea when combined with antihistamines or corticosteroids without added side effects.

Onset of action was within one hour in common cold studies. There was no rebound in rhinorrhea following discontinuation of ipratropium. The drug maintains its effectiveness in long-term use, and may reduce the need for concomitant rhinitis medications. Ipratropium does not cause systemic anticholinergic side effects when topically administered. Dryness of the nose and mouth may be encountered, but can be controlled with a reduction in dosage.

Ipratropium nasal spray comes in two strengths: 0.03% for chronic therapy in allergic and nonallergic rhinitis, and 0.06% for acute therapy in the common cold. It is the only approved prescription nasal spray for the control of rhinorrhea in colds. It has been helpful in other refractory conditions as well, such as gustatory rhinitis (Table 6.7).

## Ocular Therapy

As mentioned in the discussion of diagnosis, ocular itching and watering nearly always accompany nasal symptoms in allergic rhinitis. In contrast to the safety of intranasal steroid use, topical ocular steroid use is hazardous due to the risk of ocular infection and cataracts. One of the reasons oral antihistamines are usually included in treatment is to control ocular itching. Topical antihistamines such as pheniramine maleate are available in combination with the vasoconstrictor naphazoline for temporary relief of eye symptoms. There is systemic absorption of the vasoconstrictor which should be avoided in severe cardiovascular disease. The antihistamine levocabastine hydrochloride is available for topical use and has compared favorably with oral terfenadine in control of ocular itching. The effect of levocabastine is immediate in contrast to cromolyn or lodoxamide which may take several days to be effective. Transient stinging of the eyes is a problem as with many ocular medications. The preservative benzalkonium chloride can damage contact lenses.

Lodoxamide is similar to cromolyn sodium, but has been released only for use in vernal keratoconjunctivitis. Cromolyn sodium ophthalmic drops are effective in reducing ocular itching, inflammation and discharge. The recommended frequency of use is 4 to 6 times per day. Full effect of the drug may not be seen for a week or more. A nonsteroidal anti-inflammatory drug, ketorolac, has also been released for treatment of allergic conjunctivitis. Four-times-a-day dosing is recommended, and ocular irritation is common. The need for frequent dosing and the common transient irritation of the eyes from the current topical ocular treatments lead to consideration of the severity of eye symptoms in the decision to start immunotherapy for the prevention of both ocular and nasal symptoms. Table 6.8 lists the available ocular agents.

| TABLE 6.8 — OCULAR AGENTS ||
|---|---|
| **Generic Drug Name** | **Trade Name** |
| Levocabastine | Livostin |
| Ketorolac | Acular |
| Lodoxamide | Alomide |
| Cromolyn sodium | Crolom 4% |

## Pregnancy and Asthma/Allergy Medications

The Food and Drug Administration has published guidelines for prescribing asthma/allergy medications to pregnant women. Drugs are classified into four groups (groups A through D) based on the available data on the relative risk. Most asthma and allergy medications are classified as group B or C. The drugs classified as group D should not be prescribed to pregnant asthmatics, including:
- Tetracycline
- Iodide-containing expectorants

These medications and FDA risk factor ratings are summarized in Tables 6.9 and 6.10.

## TABLE 6.9 — RISK TO FETUS OF ALLERGY AND ASTHMA MEDICATIONS DURING PREGNANCY

| | Risk Factor Category |
|---|---|
| **Bronchodilator** | |
| Ipratropium | B |
| Terbutaline | B |
| Albuterol | C |
| Metaproterenol | C |
| Salmeterol | C |
| Theophylline | C |
| **Anti-inflammatory** | |
| Cromolyn sodium | B |
| Nedocromil sodium | B |
| Beclomethasone dipropionate | C |
| Budesonide | C |
| Flunisolide | C |
| Fluticasone | C |
| Triamcinolone | C |
| Dexamethasone | (Not rated) |
| Prednisone | (Not rated) |
| **Antihistamine** | |
| Cetirizine | B |
| Chlorpheniramine | B |
| Loratadine | B |
| Triprolidine | B |
| Astemizole | C |
| Brompheniramine | C |
| Terfenadine | C |

### Key to Risk Factor Ratings
(According to Manufacturer's FDA Approved Product Labeling)

**A**    **Controlled studies show no risk.** Adequate, well-controlled studies in pregnant women have failed to demonstrate risk to the fetus.

**B**    **No evidence of risk in humans.** Either animal findings show risk, but human findings do not; if no adequate human studies have been done, animal findings are negative.

**C**    **Risk cannot be ruled out.** Human studies are lacking, animal studies are either positive for fetal risk, or lacking as well. However, potential benefits may justify potential risk.

**D**    **Positive evidence of risk.**

**X**    **Contraindicated in pregnancy.**

Modified from: National Asthma Education Program: expert panel report. *Guidelines for the Diagnosis and Management of Asthma.* Bethesda, MD: National Institutes of Health; 1991:127.

## TABLE 6.10—RISK OF ALLERGY AND ASTHMA MEDICATIONS IN FIRST TRIMESTER OF PREGNANCY

| Drug | No. of Patients Exposed | Standardized Risk* | Significance |
|---|---|---|---|
| Corticosteroids | 145 | 0.67 | |
| Tripelennamine | 100 | 0.81 | |
| Isoproterenol | 31 | 0.94 | |
| Atropine | 401 | 1.04 | |
| Ephedrine | 373 | 1.07 | |
| Chlorpheniramine | 1,070 | 1.20 | |
| Diphenhydramine | 595 | 1.25 | |
| Phenylephrine | 1,249 | 1.31 | <0.05 |
| Theophylline | 117 | 1.38 | |
| Phenylpropanolamine | 726 | 1.40 | <0.01 |
| Hydroxyzine | 50 | 1.44 | |
| Epinephrine | 189 | 1.71 | <0.05 |
| Brompheniramine | 65 | 2.34 | <0.05 |

* Normalized risk is 1.00.

Reproduced from: National Asthma Education Program: expert panel report. *Guidelines for the Diagnosis and Management of Asthma.* Bethesda, MD: National Institute of Health; 1991:126.

# 7 Immunotherapy

Immunotherapy is for those patients with allergic rhinitis and conjunctivitis who cannot adequately control their symptoms using antihistamines and nasal steroid sprays. For a patient with isolated allergy to ragweed, immunotherapy is usually not needed since the season lasts only a few weeks of the year.

Most allergic rhinitis patients are sensitive to multiple pollens. A patient sensitive to tree, grass and weed pollens has symptoms for 6 to 9 months of the year. In some parts of the country, grass season extends throughout the year. Other allergic patients have been sensitized to dust mites as well as pollens. For these patients, immunotherapy provides relief from nearly year-round symptoms with much less need for medication. When used for correctly selected patients, immunotherapy provides 80% of the patients treated with 50% to 75% relief from their allergic rhinitis and conjunctivitis symptoms. Immunotherapy using pollen, house-dust mite, cat, and some mold extracts reduces symptoms and sensitivity to nasal or bronchial provocation.

The beneficial response to immunotherapy is dose related. Since doses near to maximum toleration are needed to produce benefit, local reactions at the site of injection are common and systemic reactions are always a possibility. Any facility giving allergy shots needs to be prepared to treat reactions, including anaphylaxis.

Part of the immunologic response to immunotherapy is the production of IgG specific antibody to the allergen injected. One of the theories of mechanisms of action of immunotherapy is that the newly generated IgG does not fix to mast cells but can react with antigen diffusing into tissues. The immunoglobulin G (IgG) response to immunotherapy develops slowly, reaching a maximum after 8 months of shots. Allergy shots are given in gradually increasing doses as tolerance for the allergen increases. By the time the maintenance dose is reached, the patient tolerates environmental exposure to the allergen as well. Maintenance shots are continued at intervals of every 2 to 4 weeks throughout the year. Allergic patients are continued on the shots until they have had 2 seasons essentially free of rhinitis and conjunctivitis symptoms. The goal of pharmacologic therapy and immunotherapy is to allow patients with allergic rhinitis to enjoy normal activities indoors and outdoors with a minimum of symptoms.

# PART 4

## REFERENCES

# 8 References

**Anticholinergics**

Baroody F, Majchel A, Roecker M, et al. Ipratropium bromide (Atrovent® Nasal Spray) reduces the nasal response to methacholine. *J Allergy Clin Immunol*. 1992;89:1065-1075.

Baroody F, Ford S, Lichtenstein LM, et al. Physiologic responses and histamine release after nasal antigen challenge: effect of atropine. *Am J Respir Crit Care Med*. 1994;149:1457-1465.

Bronsky EA, Druce H, Findlay SR, et al. A clinical trial of ipratropium bromide nasal spray in patients with perennial nonallergic rhinitis. *J Allergy Clin Immunol*. 1995;95:1117-1122.

Grossman J, Banov C, Boggs P, et al. Use of ipratropium bromide nasal spray in chronic treatment of nonallergic perennial rhinitis, alone and in combination with other perennial rhinitis medications. *J Allergy Clin Immunol*. 1995;95:1123-1127.

Meltzer EO, Orgel HA, Bronsky EA, et al. Ipratropium bromide aqueous nasal spray for patients with perennial allergic rhinitis: a study of its effect on their symptoms, quality of life, and nasal cytology. *J Allergy Clin Immunol*. 1992;90:242-249.

**Antihistamines**

Barnes CL, McKenzie CA, Webster KD, Poinsett-Holmes K. Cetirizine: a new nonsedating antihistamine. *Ann Pharmacother*. 1993;27:464-470.

Bronsky E, Boggs P, Findlay S, et al. Comparative efficacy and safety of a once-daily loratadine-pseudoephedrine combination versus its components alone and placebo in the management of seasonal allergic rhinitis. *J Allergy Clin Immunol*. 1995;96: 139-147.

Busse WW. Role of antihistamines in allergic disease. *Ann Allergy*. 1994;72:371-375.

Honig PK, Wortham DC, Zamani K, et al. Terfenadine-ketoconazole interaction: pharmacokinetic and electrocardiographic consequences. *JAMA*. 1993; 269:1513-1518.

Monahan BP, Ferguson CL, Killeary ES, et al. Torsade de pointes occurring in association with terfenadine use. *JAMA*. 1990; 264:2788-2790.

Simon FE, Simon KJ. The pharmacology and use of $H_1$-receptor antagonist drugs. *N Eng J Med*. 1994;330:1663-1670.

Simons FER, McMillan JL, Simons KJ. A double-blind, single-dose, crossover comparison of cetirizine, terfenadine, loratadine, astemizole and chlorpheniramine versus placebo: suppressive effects on histamine-induced wheals and flares during 24 hours in normal subjects. *J Allergy Clin Immunol*. 1990;86:540-547.

Tobin JR, Doyle TP, Ackerman AD, et al. Astemizole-induced cardiac conduction disturbances in a child. *JAMA*. 1991;226: 2734-2740.

Woosley RL, Chen Y, Freiman JP, et al. Mechanism of the cardiotoxic actions of terfenadine. *JAMA*. 1993;269:1532-1536.

## Avoidance

Platts-Mills TAE. Allergen avoidance at home: what really works *J Respir Dis*. 1989;10:53-55.

Platts-Mills TAE, Mitchell EB, Chapman MD, Heymann PW. Dust mite allergy: its clinical significance. *Hosp Pract*. 1987;22:91-100.

Solomon WR, Bruge HA, Boise JR. Exclusion of particulate allergens by window air conditioners. *J Allergy Clin Immunol*. 1980;65:305-308.

## Decongestants

Bronsky E, Boggs P, Findlay S, et al. Comparative efficacy and safety of a once-daily loratadine-pseudoephedrine combination versus its components alone and placebo in the management of seasonal allergic rhinitis. *J Allergy Clin Immunol*. 1995;96: 139-147.

Hamilton LH, Chobanian SL, Cato A, et al. A study of sustained action pseudoephedrine in allergic rhinitis. *Ann Allergy*. 1982;48:87-92.

Pentel P. Toxicity of over-the-counter stimulants. *JAMA*. 1984; 252:1898-1903.

**General**

Druce HM, Hanifin JM, Meltzer EO, et al. Histamine-induced disease: impact of new research on treatment algorithms. *J Respir Dis*. 1992;13 (suppl):S1-S39.

Kaliner M, Lemanske R. Rhinitis and asthma. *JAMA*. 1992; 268:2807-2829.

Mathews KP. Respiratory atopic disease. *JAMA*. 1982;248:2587-2610.

Meltzer EO. An overview of current pharmacotherapy in perennial rhinitis. *J Allergy Clin Immunol*. 1995;95:1097-1110.

Naclerio RM. Allergic rhinitis. *N Eng J Med*. 1991; 325:860-869.

National Asthma Education Program: expert panel report. *Guidelines for the Diagnosis and Management of Asthma*. Bethesda, MD: National Institutes of Health; 1991:66.

Nelson HS. Diagnostic procedures in allergy. *Ann Allergy*. 1983;51:411-416.

Norman PS. Allergic rhinitis. *J Allergy Clin Immunol*. 1985; 75:531-545.

Ten RM, Klein JS, Frigas E. Allergy skin testing. *Mayo Clin Proc*. 1995;70:783-784.

Van Arsdel PP, Larson EB. Diagnostic tests for patients with suspected allergic disease. *Ann Intern Med*. 1989;110:304-312.

White MV, Kaliner MA. Mediators of allergic rhinitis. *J Allergy Clin Immunol*. 1992;90:699-704.

**Immunotherapy**

Fortner BR, Dantzler BS, Tipton WR, et al. The effect of weekly versus monthly ragweed allergen injections on immunological parameters. *Ann Allergy*. 1981;47:147-150.

Greenberg MA, Kaufman CR, Gonzalez GE, et al. Late and immediate systemic-allergic reactions to inhalant allergen immunotherapy. *J Allergy Clin Immunol*. 1986;77:865-870.

Metzger WJ, Turner E, Patterson R. The safety of immunotherapy during pregnancy. *J Allergy Clin Immunol*. 1978;61:268-272.

Nelson HS. Diagnostic procedures in allergy: I. allergy skin testing. *Ann Allergy*. 1983;51:411-416.

Norman PS. Immunotherapy for nasal allergy. *J Allergy Clin Immunol*. 1988;81:992-996.

## Nasal Corticosteroids

Fluticasone propionate nasal spray for allergic rhinitis. *Medical Letter*. 1995;37:5-6.

Intranasal budesonide for allergic rhinitis. *Medical Letter*. 1994;36:63-64.

Juniper EF, Kline PA, Hargreave FE, et al. Comparison of beclomethasone dipropionate aqueous nasal spray, astemizole, and the combination in the prophylactic treatment of ragweed pollen-induced rhino-conjunctivitis. *J Allergy Clin Immunol*. 1989; 83:627-633.

Knight A, Kolin A. Long-term efficacy and safety of beclomethasone dipropionate aerosol in perennial rhinitis. *Ann Allergy*. 1983;50:81-84.

Norman PS, Winkenwerder WL, Agbayani BF, et al. Adrenal function during the use of dexamethasone aerosols in the treatment of ragweed hay fever. *J Allergy*. 1967;40:67-61.

Siegel SC. Topical intranasal corticosteroid therapy in rhinitis. *J Allergy Cin Immunol*. 1988;81:984-991.

Simpson RJ. Budesonide and terfenadine, separately and in combination, in the treatment of hay fever. *Ann Allergy*. 1994;73:497-502.

Storms W, Bronsky E, Findlay S, et al. Once daily triamcinolone acetonide nasal spray is effective for the treatment of perennial allergic rhinitis. *Ann Allergy*. 1991;66:329-334.

van Bavel J, Findlay SR, Hampel FC, et al. Intranasal fluticasone propionate is more effective than terfenadine tablets for seasonal allergic rhinitis. *Arch Intern Med*. 1994;154:2699-2704.

## Ocular Therapy

Bahmer FA, Ruprecht KW. Safety and efficacy of topical levocabastine compared with oral terfenadine. *Ann Allergy*. 1994;72:429-434.

Cromolyn sodium for allergic conjunctivitis. *Medical Letter*. 1985;27:7-8.

Ketorolac for seasonal allergic conjunctivitis. *Medical Letter*. 1993;35:88-89

Ophthalmic levocabastine for allergic conjunctivitis. *Medical Letter*. 1994;36:35-36.

**Sinusitis and Nasal Polyps**

Kennedy DW. Functional endoscopic sinus surgery techniques. *Arch Otolaryngol*. 1985;111:643-649.

Lildholdt T, Fogstrup J, Gammelgaard N, et al. Surgical versus medical treatment of nasal polyps. *Acta Otolaryngol*. 1988;105:140-143.

Rachelefsky GS, Katz RM, Siegel SC. Chronic sinus disease with associated reactive airway disease in children. *Pediatrics*. 1984;73:526-529.

Settipane GA, Chafee FH. Nasal polyps in asthma and rhinitis: a review of 6,037 patients. *J Allergy Clin Immunol*. 1977;59:1721.

Slavin RG. Recalcitrant asthma: could sinusitis be the culprit? *J Respir Dis*. 1991;12:182-194.

Slavin RG. Relationship of nasal disease and sinusitis to bronchial asthma. *Ann Allergy*. 1982;49: 76-80.

Williams JW, Simel DL, Roberts L, Samsa GP. Clinical evaluation for sinusitis. *Ann Intern Med*. 1992; 117:705-710.

# Index

Note: Page numbers in *italics* indicate figures; page numbers followed by *t* indicate tables.

Acute rhinitis, 13
Adenoid(s), 16
Age
　allergic rhinitis onset and, 29
　otitis and, 36
Albuterol, 76t
Alkylamine(s), 60t
Allergen(s)
　environmental, seasonal, 20t, 28-29
　indoor, 56, 56t
　potency of, in intradermal extracts, 34-35
Allergic response
　components of, 19
　immediate, 23
　late-phase, 23-24
Allergic rhinitis
　animal exposure and, 28
　atopic dermatitis in, 28
　autonomic nervous system in, 23
　bronchial asthma with, antihistamine contraindication in, 64
　causes of, 14t
　conditions associated with, 15t
　differential diagnosis of, 30t, 37
　ELISA in, 35
　familial, 28
　history taking in, 27-29
　incidence of, 13
　inflammatory cascade in, 19, *22*
　laboratory tests in, 31-32
　molds in, 29
　nasal mucosa in, 19, 31
　onset age in, 29
　perennial. *See* Perennial rhinitis.
　physical examination in, 30-31
　progression of, to sinusitis, 37
　provocation testing in, 36
　ragweed and, 13
　RAST testing in, 35
　seasonal variation in, 28-29
　skin testing in, 33-35
　substance P and, 23
　symptoms of, 14t, 27-28

treatment of, 15t
  immunotherapy in, 23, 79-80
  in pregnancy, 74, 76t-77t
Allergy unit, 34
Animal(s), as allergens, 28
Anticholinergic(s)
  action mechanism of, 71
  antihistamines as, 63
  effectiveness of, 59t, 73
Antigen(s), 19
Antihistamine(s)
  action mechanisms of, 57
  anticholinergic effects of, 63
  cardiac effects of, 63-64
  classification of, 59, 60t-61t
  in co-existent allergic rhinitis and bronchial asthma, 64
  dosage of, 60t-61t
  duration of, 59, 62
  effectiveness of, 59t
  in pregnancy, 76t
  sedation from, 62-63
  for sinusitis, 47
  skin testing and, 32
  trade names for, 60t-61t
Arachidonic acid metabolism, products of, *22*, 23
Aspirin, 17
Astemizole
  appetite stimulation and, 63
  cardiac effects of, 63-64
  contraindications to, 63-64
  dosage of, 60t
  duration of, 62
  in pregnancy, 76t
Asthma
  aspirin sensitivity in, 17
  nasal passage disorders in, 17
Audiometry, 37
Autonomic nervous system, 23
Azatadine maleate, 60t
Azelastine, 72t

Beclomethasone, 58t
  in pregnancy, 76t
  relative potency of, 71t
  trade names and dosages of, 70t
Birth control pill(s), 16
Bony spur, septal, *51*

Bradykinin, *22*, 23
Brompheniramine
  dosage of, 60t
  duration of, 62
  in pregnancy, 76t-77t
Bronchial asthma, allergic rhinitis with, antihistamine contraindication in, 64
Bronchial provocation testing, 36
Bronchodilator(s), 76t
Budesonide, 58t
  in pregnancy, 76t
  trade name and dosage of, 70t

Cardiac arrhythmia, 63
Cetirizine
  for bronchospasm, 64
  dosage of, 60t
  duration of, 62
  in pregnancy, 76t
  sedation from, 63
Chlorpheniramine
  dosage of, 60t
  duration of, 62
  in pregnancy, 76t-77t
Chronic rhinitis. *See also* Allergic rhinitis.
  causes of, 14t
  symptoms of, 14t
  treatment of, 15t
    anticholinergics in, 71-73
    antihistamines in, 57, 58t-59t, 59, 60t-61t, 62-64
    avoidance of responsible allergens in, 55-56
    cromolyn sodium in, 71
    decongestants in, 64-65
    goals of, 11, 55
    immunotherapy in, 79-80
    miscellaneous agents in, 72t
    ocular, 73, 75
    pharmacologic, 58t
    in pregnancy, 74, 76t-77t
Chymase, 20, *22*
Ciliary dyskinesia, 30t
Clemastine fumarate, 60t
Complications of rhinitis
  otitis as, 36-37
  sinusitis as. *See* Sinusitis.
Computed tomography, of sinuses, 41-43, *43-45*
Concha bullosa, 13

Corticosteroid(s). *See also* Steroid(s); Steroid nasal spray.
  action mechanism of, 65, 69
  for allergic response, 24
  for nasal polyps, 17, 47
  in pregnancy, 77t
  relative potencies of, 71t
  skin testing and, 32
Cranial penetration, of sinus infection, 47
Cromolyn sodium, 58t
  for allergic response, 24
  effectiveness of, 59t
  indications for, 71
  in pregnancy, 76t
  trade name and dosage for, 72t
Cycloxygenase, *22*, 23
Cyproheptadine hydrochloride, 60t
Cystic fibrosis, 13

Decongestant(s). *See also* Decongestant nasal spray.
  contraindications to, 65
  effectiveness of, 59t
  side effects of, 65
  for sinusitis, 47
  trade names for, 68t
  withdrawal from, 65
Decongestant nasal spray
  action mechanism of, 64
  chronic use of, 16, 65
  dosages of, 66t-68t
  trade names of, 66t-68t
Dexamethasone, 58t
  trade name and dosage of, 70t
Diphenhydramine
  dosage of, 60t
  in pregnancy, 77t
Dust mite(s), 29
  control measures for, 56, 56t

Eczema, 28
Electrolyte abnormality, 64
Endoscopic view
  of acute purulent sinusitis, *34*
  of nasal polyp, *33*
  of right uncinate process, *42*
Environmental allergen(s), seasonal, 20t
Enzyme-linked immunosorbent assay (ELISA), 35
Eosinophil
  count of, 31

in immediate allergic response, 24
inflammation of, 37
mast cell degranulation and, 20, *22*
Eosinophilic hypertrophic sinusitis, nasal polyps and, 17
Eosinophilic nonallergic rhinitis. *See* NARES.
Ephedrine, 58t
 dosage of, 66t
 in pregnancy, 77t
Epinephrine, 58t
 in pregnancy, 77t
Ethanolamine, 60t
Ethmoid air cell, 40
Ethylenediamine, 60t
Eye(s). *See also* Ocular *entries*.
 itching and watering of
  in allergic rhinitis, 37
  treatment of, 73, 75

Family, allergic rhinitis in, 28
Fexofenadine, 60t
Flunisolide, 58t
 in pregnancy, 76t
 relative potency of, 71t
 trade names and dosages of, 70t
Fluticasone, 58t
 relative potency of, 71t
 trade name and dosage of, 70t

Gustatory rhinitis, causes of, 16

Headache
 in allergic rhinitis, 27-28
 sinus-related, 40
Hearing loss, 36
Histamine
 mast cell degranulation and, 20, *22*
 nasal itching and, 23
 sneezing and, 23
History taking, 27-28
House dust mite(s), 29
 control measures for, 56, 56t
Humoral evaluation, 44-46
Hydrocortisone, 71t
Hydroxyzine
 dosage of, 60t
 duration of, 62
 in pregnancy, 77t

Hyperactive nose, 16
Hypogammaglobulinemia, 46
Hypothyroidism, 16

Immune deficiency, 44-46
Immunoglobulin E, antigen-specific
  detection of, 32
  formation of, 19
Immunologic mechanism(s), in nasal mucosa, *21*
Immunotherapy
  allergen potency in, 35
  for allergic rhinitis, 23
  dose response in, 79
  effectiveness of, 79
  indications for, 79
  mechanisms of, 79-80
*In vitro* testing, in allergic rhinitis, 35
Indoor allergen(s), 29
Inflammatory cascade
  in allergic rhinitis, *22*
  steps in, 19
Interleukin(s), 19-20, *22*, 23
Ipratropium, 58t
  duration of, 73
  effectiveness of, 71-73
  in pregnancy, 76t
  trade name and dosage for, 72t
Isoproterenol, 77t

Ketorolac, 74, 74t

Laboratory testing, 31-32
Leukotriene(s)
  in inflammatory cascade, *22*, 23
  sneezing and, 23
Levocabastine, 74, 74t
Lipoxygenase, *22*, 23
Liver disease, 63
Lodoxamide, 74, 75t
Loratadine
  dosage of, 60t
  duration of, 62
  in pregnancy, 76t
  sedative effects of, 62-63

Mast cell(s)
  newly generated mediators and, 20, *22*

preformed products of, 20, *22*
substance P and, 23
Maxillary sinus
  air fluid level in, *46*
  chronic infection in, 39
  opacification of, *47, 49*
  polyp in, *50*
  size of, *48*
Metaproterenol, 76t
Middle ear pressure, equalization of, 37
Mold, 29

Naphazoline, 58t, 72
  dosage of, 66t
NARES
  causes of, 14t
  conditions associated with, 15t
  nasal mucosa in, 31
  symptoms of, 14t, 16
  treatment of, 15t
Nasal congestion
  after allergen challenge, 23
  anatomy and, 13, 16
  pathophysiology of, 23
Nasal itching, 23
Nasal mucosa
  immunological mechanisms in, *21*
  inflammation of, 31
  in NARES, 31
Nasal patency, 31
Nasal polyp, 13
  asthma with, 17
  causes of, 14t
  chronic sinusitis and, 38, 43-44
  computed tomography of, *50*
  conditions associated with, 15t
  corticosteroids for, 17
  endoscopic view of, *33*
  onset age in, 29
  physical examination of, 30
  recurrence of, 44
  steroid nasal spray for, 47
  symptoms of, 14t
  treatment of, 15t
Nasal provocation testing, 36
Nedocromil sodium, 76t
Neuroblastoma, *52*

Neutrophil(s), 24
Neutrophilic rhinosinusitis, 14t-15t
Nonallergic rhinitis with eosinophilia syndrome. *See* NARES.
Nose. *See also* Nasal *entries*.
 physical examination of, 31

Ocular penetration, of sinus infection, 47
Ocular therapy, 73, 75
Ostiomeatal complex
 infection of, 39
 normal, *38*
 obstruction and secondary sinusitis of, 38-39, *39*
Otitis
 age and, 36
 diagnosis of, 36
 hypogammaglobulinemia and, 46
 physical examination in, 37
 treatment of, 37
Oxymetazoline, 58t
 dosage of, 67t

Perennial rhinitis
 asthma with, 17
 skin testing in, 29
Phenothiazine(s), 60t
Phenylephrine, 58t
 dosage of, 66t-67t
 in pregnancy, 77t
Phenylpropanolamine, 58t
 in pregnancy, 77t
Piperazine(s), 60t
Platelet activating factor, *22*, 23
Pneumonia, 46
Pollen
 indoor, control of, 56
 seasonal variation in, 28-29
Polymorphonuclear leukocyte, 31-32
Polyp, nasal. *See* Nasal polyp.
Prednisone, 76t
Pregnancy
 allergy and asthma medications in, 74, 76t-77t
 nasal congestion in, 16
 rhinitis in, 30t
Prick test, 34
Promethazine, 60t
Prostaglandin(s)
 in inflammatory cascade, *22*, 23

nasal itching and, 23
Protein nitrogen unit, 34-35
Provocation testing, 36
Pseudoephedrine, 58t
  dosage of, 68t

Q-T interval, 63

Radioallergosorbent (RAST) test, 35
Radiography of sinuses, 41, *46-47, 49*
  in asthma, 17
Rhinitis, differential diagnosis of, 30t
Rhinitis medicamentosa
  causes of, 14t
  conditions associated with, 15t
  decongestant spray and, 16
  differential diagnosis of, 30t
  symptoms of, 14t
  treatment of, 15t
Rhinorrhea, 23
Rhinoscopy, 30-31
Rhinosinusitis, neutrophilic, 14t-15t

Salmeterol, 76t
Seasonal variation
  in environmental allergens, 20t
  in pollens, 28-29
Sedation, 62-63
Septum
  bony spur in, *51*
  deformity of, 13
    differential diagnosis of, 30t
    nasal congestion and, 13
  neuroblastoma of, *52*
Sinus
  air fluid level in, *46*
  computed tomography of, *43-45*
  obstruction of, 40
  opacification of, *47, 49*
  radiography of, 41, *46-47, 49*
Sinus headache, 40
Sinusitis
  acute
    pathogens in, 40
    symptoms of, 40
  acute bacterial
    diagnosis of, 37

    differential diagnosis of, 37
    in viral rhinitis, 37
  acute purulent, endoscopic view of, *34*
  antibiotics for, 42-43
  bilateral, *45*
  chronic
    eosinophilic inflammation in, 37
    ethmoid air cells in, 40
    hypogammaglobulinemia and, 46
    inhalant allergies and, 37
    nasal polyps in, 38
    pathogens in, 41
    pathophysiology of, 39-40
    symptoms of, 41
  computed tomography in, 41-43, *45*
  cranial/orbital penetration of infection from, 47
  decongestants for, 47
  establishment of normal mucus drainage in, 47
  immune deficiency and, 44-46
  maxillary cavities in, 39
  nasal polyps and, 38, 43-44
  ostiomeatal complex in, 38-39, *38-39*
  physical examination in, 41
  purulent, 41
  surgical treatment of, 44, 47
Skin testing
  advantages of, 32
  antihistamines and, 32
  after cessation of allergy, 35, *36*
  contraindications to, 32
  corticosteroids and, 32
  extract potency in, 34-35
  interpretation of, 34
  materials for, 32
  nasal polyps and, 17
  in perennial rhinitis, 29
  procedures in, 33-34
Sneezing, 23
Steroid(s). *See* Corticosteroid(s); Steroid nasal spray.
Steroid nasal spray
  dosage of, 69
  effectiveness of, 59t
  safety of, 69
  side effects of, 69
  systemic effects of, 69
  trade names and dosages of, 70t
Structural rhinitis, 14t-15t

Substance P, 23

Terbutaline, 76t
Terfenadine, 74
  cardiac effects of, 63-64
  contraindications to, 63-64
  dosage of, 60t
  duration of, 62
  in pregnancy, 76t
Tetrahydrozoline, 58t
  dosage of, 67t
Theophylline, in pregnancy, 76t-77t
Torsade de pointes, 63
Triamcinolone, 58t
  in pregnancy, 76t
  relative potency of, 71t
  trade name and dosage of, 70t
Tripelennamine
  dosage of, 60t
  in pregnancy, 78t
Triprolidine, 76t
Tryptase, 20, *22*
Tumor necrosis factor alpha, *22*, 23
Turbinate(s), 13
Tympanometry, 37

Uncinate process, endoscopic view of, *42*

Vasomotor rhinitis
  causes of, 14t
  conditions associated with, 15t
  differential diagnosis of, 30t
  symptoms of, 14t, 16
  treatment of, 15t
Viral rhinitis
  acute bacterial sinusitis in, 37
  course of, 13
  differential diagnosis of, 37
  symptoms of, 13

Wegener's granulomatosis, 30t

Xylometazoline, 58t
  dosage of, 67t